Manual of Practical
# Medical Biochemistry

# Manual of Practical
# Medical Biochemistry

*(As per the Revised Competency Based NMC/MCI Curriculum)*

## Third Edition

**Evangeline Jones** MD
*Formerly* Professor and Head
Department of Biochemistry
Vinayaka Missions Kirupanandha
Variyar Medical College

and

Government Mohan Kumaramangalam Medical College
Salem, Tamil Nadu, India

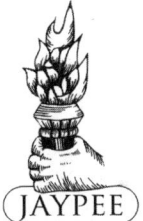

**JAYPEE BROTHERS MEDICAL PUBLISHERS**
*The Health Sciences Publisher*
New Delhi | London

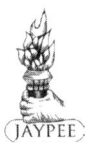

**Jaypee Brothers Medical Publishers (P) Ltd**

**Headquarters**

Jaypee Brothers Medical Publishers (P) Ltd
EMCA House, 23/23-B
Ansari Road, Daryaganj
New Delhi - 110 002, India
Landline: +91-11-23272143, +91-11-23272703,
+91-11-23282021, +91-11-23245672
Email: jaypee@jaypeebrothers.com

**Corporate Office**

Jaypee Brothers Medical Publishers (P) Ltd
4838/24, Ansari Road, Daryaganj
New Delhi 110 002, India
Phone: +91-11-43574357
Fax: +91-11-43574314
Email: jaypee@jaypeebrothers.com

**Overseas Office**

J.P. Medical Ltd
83 Victoria Street, London
SW1H 0HW (UK)
Phone: +44 20 3170 8910
Fax: +44 (0)20 3008 6180
Email: info@jpmedpub.com

Website: www.jaypeebrothers.com
Website: www.jaypeedigital.com

© 2022, Jaypee Brothers Medical Publishers

The views and opinions expressed in this book are solely those of the original contributor(s)/author(s) and do not necessarily represent those of editor(s) of the book.

All rights reserved. No part of this publication may be reproduced, stored or transmitted in any form or by any means, electronic, mechanical, photocopying, recording or otherwise, without the prior permission in writing of the publishers/editors.

All brand names and product names used in this book are trade names, service marks, trademarks or registered trademarks of their respective owners. The publisher is not associated with any product or vendor mentioned in this book.

Medical knowledge and practice change constantly. This book is designed to provide accurate, authoritative information about the subject matter in question. However, readers are advised to check the most current information available on procedures included and check information from the manufacturer of each product to be administered, to verify the recommended dose, formula, method and duration of administration, adverse effects and contraindications. It is the responsibility of the practitioner to take all appropriate safety precautions. Neither the publisher nor the author(s)/editor(s) assume any liability for any injury and/or damage to persons or property arising from or related to use of material in this book.

This book is sold on the understanding that the publisher is not engaged in providing professional medical services. If such advice or services are required, the services of a competent medical professional should be sought.

Every effort has been made where necessary to contact holders of copyright to obtain permission to reproduce copyright material. If any have been inadvertently overlooked, the publisher will be pleased to make the necessary arrangements at the first opportunity.

**Inquiries for bulk sales may be solicited at:** jaypee@jaypeebrothers.com

*Manual of Practical Medical Biochemistry*

*First Edition: 2011*
*Second Edition: 2016*
*Third Edition:* **2022**

ISBN: 978-93-5465-510-4

*Printed at: Sterling Graphics Pvt. Ltd.*

## Dedicated to

*Almighty God*
*For His grace and guidance*

# Preface to the Third Edition

This edition of the laboratory manual in biochemistry has been revised as per the *Competency based Undergraduate Curriculum for the Medical Graduate* issued by the *Medical Council of India/National Medical Council.*

*Manual of Practical Medical Biochemistry* has been updated keeping in line with the guidelines and maintaining a clear focus of teaching the first-year medical students, the art of practical medical biochemistry. The revised edition has become necessary in view of the changing trends in the teaching methodology and learning processes. Keeping this in mind, changes have been made throughout this edition, adding details of latest equipments, procedures and laboratory requirements which are mandatory now. Updated Clinical Case studies and Objective Structured Practical Examination (OSPE) and other integrated topics are the highlights of this manual.

I would like to acknowledge with gratitude the help rendered by my friends and teaching colleagues of the Institutions where I had worked earlier—Department of Biochemistry, Vinayaka Missions Kirupanandha Variyar Medical College and Government Mohan Kumaramangalam Medical College Medical College, Salem, Tamil Nadu, India.

At this juncture, I would like to thank my teachers of Biochemistry, whose advice has encouraged me in compiling this book. I also thank my husband Dr P Jones Ronald, Nephrologist for his continuous encouragement and contribution by way of drawing the diagrams in this manual. I thank M/s Jaypee Brothers Medical Publishers (P) Ltd, New Delhi, for bringing up this book tidily and on time.

I hope and wish that this manual will be useful for the students of medical, dental and allied medical sciences in understanding the beauty that underlies the basis of Practical Biochemistry.

**Evangeline Jones**

# Preface to the First Edition

The laboratory manual in biochemistry is based on the practical work schedule allotted to the first year MBBS students as per the guidelines issued by the Medical Council of India (MCI).

This book *Manual of Practical Medical Biochemistry* has been compiled in simple language with a clear focus on equipping the medical students, the clinical aspects of practical biochemistry.

I would like to acknowledge with gratitude the help rendered by all the staff of the Department of Biochemistry, Government Mohan Kumaramangalam Medical College, Salem, Tamil Nadu, India, in bringing out the manual, especially my erstwhile colleagues in the Department; Dr R Nagendran MD and Dr Priya Jeyapal MD—Professors of Biochemistry, for their constructive suggestions, and Mrs CR Jamuna BSc, for her help in preparing and typing the manuscript. I thank my husband Dr P Jones Ronald MD DM, Nephrologist, for his continuous encouragement and contribution by way of drawing the diagrams in this manual.

I hope and wish that this manual will be useful for the students of medical, dental and allied medical sciences in understanding the beauty that underlies the basis of biochemistry.

**Evangeline Jones**

# Contents

## 1. GENERAL

1. **General Instructions** .................................................................................................3
   - Biochemistry Practicals: General Instructions to the Students    3

2. **Laboratory Equipments and Procedures** ...............................................................4
   - A. Commonly Used Laboratory Equipments    4
   - B. Good Safe Laboratory Procedures and Safety Rules    8
   - C. Laboratory Waste Disposal    9
   - D. Collection and Handling of Samples    11

3. **Buffers and pH** ............................................................................................................13
   - Preparation of Buffers and Estimation of pH    13

4. **Quality Control** ..........................................................................................................16
   - Quality Control    16

## 2. ANALYSIS OF URINE AND CEREBROSPINAL FLUID

5. **Normal Urine: Characteristics and Analysis** ........................................................21
   - Normal Urine    21
   - Specimen Collection    21
   - Physical Characteristics    21
   - Chemical Characteristics    23
   - Analysis of Normal Urine    25

6. **Abnormal Constituents of Urine** .............................................................................28
   - Abnormal Chemical Constituents of Urine    28
   - Analysis of Abnormal Constituents of Urine    31

7. **Screening of Urine for Inborn Errors of Metabolism and the Use of Paper Chromatography** ..........................................................................34
   - Screening of Urine for Inborn Errors of Metabolism (IEM)    34
   - A. Congenital Disorders of Carbohydrate Metabolism    35
   - B. Congenital Disorders of Protein Metabolism    36

8. **Composition of Cerebrospinal Fluid** ......................................................................41
   - Cerebrospinal Fluid (CSF)    41

## 3. QUANTITATIVE EXPERIMENTS

**9. Principles of Colorimetry** .......................................................................................... 45
- Colorimetry (Absorption Photometry) — 45

**10. Principles of Spectrophotometer** ............................................................................ 49
- Spectrophotometer — 49

**11. Estimation of Glucose** ............................................................................................. 51
- Demonstration and Estimation — 51

**12. Glucose Tolerance Test** ........................................................................................... 58
- Glucose Tolerance Test Curves (GTT) — 60

**13. Estimation of Serum and Urine Creatinine: Creatinine Clearance** ......................... 62
- Estimation of Creatinine in Serum
  (By Alkaline Picrate Method—Based on Jaffe's Reaction) — 62
- Estimation of Creatinine (Using Protein-Free Filtrate)
  (By Alkaline Picrate Method—Based on Jaffe's Method) — 64
- Creatinine in Urine and Creatinine Clearance — 66

**14. Estimation of Urea** ................................................................................................... 68
- Structure of Urea — 68
- Estimation of Urea (By Diacetyl Monoxime Method) (Using Protein-Free Filtrate) — 70

**15. Serum Proteins—Albumin: Globulin Ratio** .............................................................. 73
- Estimation of Serum Total Proteins, Albumin: Globulin (A:G) Ratio — 73

**16. Serum Total Cholesterol** .......................................................................................... 77
- Estimation of Total Cholesterol in Serum — 77

**17. Lipid Profile** .............................................................................................................. 79
- Estimation of HDL Cholesterol and Triglycerides — 79

**18. Serum Calcium and Phosphorus** ............................................................................. 82
- Estimation of Serum Calcium — 82
- Estimation of Serum Phosphorus (Inorganic) — 84

**19. Serum Bilirubin** ........................................................................................................ 87
- Estimation of Bilirubin (Demonstration) — 87

**20. Serum Transaminases** ............................................................................................. 90
- Estimation of Serum Transaminases (SGOT and SGPT) (By Reitman and Frankel method) — 90

**21. Serum Alkaline Phosphatase** ................................................................................... 92
- Estimation of Serum Alkaline Phosphatase (ALP) — 92

**22. Serum Uric Acid** ....................................................................................................... 94
- Estimation of Uric Acid in Serum — 94

Contents

## 4. EQUIPMENTS AND PROCEDURES

**23. Point of Care Testing** ....................................................................................**101**
- Point of Care Testing (POCT)     101

**24. pH Meter** .........................................................................................................**103**
- pH meter     103

**25. Paper Chromatography and Thin Layer Chromatography** ...............**105**
- Paper Chromatography (Separation of Amino Acids)     105
- Thin Layer Chromatography (TLC)     107

**26. Protein Electrophoresis** .................................................................................**108**
- Electrophoresis     108
- Paper Electrophoresis (Separation of serum proteins)     109

**27. Polyacrylamide Gel Electrophoresis** .........................................................**111**
- Polyacrylamide Gel Electrophoresis (PAGE)     111

**28. Electrolyte Analysis** ......................................................................................**113**
- Estimation of Electrolytes—By Flame Photometer     113
- Electrolyte Analysis by Ion-Selective Electrode (ISE)     114

**29. Arterial Blood Gas Analyzer** .......................................................................**118**
- ABG Analyzer (Arterial Blood Gas Analyzer)     118

**30. Enzyme-Linked Immunosorbent Assay** ..................................................**121**
- Enzyme-Linked Immunosorbent Assay (ELISA)     121

**31. Immunodiffusion** ..........................................................................................**123**
- Principle of Immunodiffusion     123

**32. Autoanalyzer** ..................................................................................................**125**
- Automated Techniques—Autoanalyzers     125

**33. DNA Isolation from Blood/Tissues** ...........................................................**128**
- DNA Isolation from Blood/Tissue     128

## 5. FUNCTION TESTS

**34. Gastric Function Tests and Analysis of Gastric Juice** ..........................**133**
- Gastric Function Tests     133

**35. Pancreatic Function Tests** ...........................................................................**137**
- Pancreatic Exocrine Function Tests     137

**36. Liver Function Tests** .....................................................................................**139**
- Liver Function Tests (LFTs)     139

## 37. Analysis of Bile .................................................................................................................. 142
- Analysis of Bile .................................................................................................. 142

## 38. Renal Function Tests ...................................................................................................... 145
- Renal Function Tests (Kidney Function Tests) ................................................... 145

## 39. Thyroid Function Tests ................................................................................................... 148
- Thyroid Function Tests ....................................................................................... 148

## 40. Adrenal Function Tests .................................................................................................. 152
- Adrenal Function Tests ....................................................................................... 152

# 6. FOOD AND ENERGY

## 41. Energy Content of Food and Glycemic Index ................................................................ 157
- Energy Content of Food ..................................................................................... 157

## 42. Fats in Food ................................................................................................................... 160
- Saturated and Unsaturated Fats in Food ............................................................ 160

# 7. CLINICAL CASE STUDIES

## 43. Basis and Rationale of Biochemical Tests Done in Certain Clinical Conditions ............................................................................................................ 165
- Basis of Biochemical Tests Done in Diseases .................................................... 165
- I. Metabolic Disorders ......................................................................................... 166
- II. Deficiency Disorders ....................................................................................... 176
- III. Inherited Disorders (Inborn Errors of Metabolism) ......................................... 179
- IV. Hormonal Disorders ....................................................................................... 183

# 8. OBJECTIVE STRUCTURED PRACTICAL EXAMINATION

## 44. Objective Structured Practical Examination ................................................................. 187
- Objective Structured Practical Examination (OSPE) .......................................... 187

# 9. REAGENTS

## 45. Reagent Preparation ..................................................................................................... 191
- Preparation of Reagents (For the Use of the Laboratory) ................................... 191
- Quantitative Estimations .................................................................................... 193

# 10. NORMAL VALUES

## 46. Normal Values ............................................................................................................... 199
- Enzyme Levels (Serum) ...................................................................................... 200

### Worksheet
Observations and Calculations ....................................................................................... 201
Index ............................................................................................................................... 211

# List of Clinically Important Cases

## CHAPTER 43—PAGES: 165–184

COMP. NO: BI11.17

| S. No | Types | Disorders | Subtypes | Pages |
|---|---|---|---|---|
| I. | Metabolic Disorders | A. Diabetes Mellitus | 1. Type–I | 166 |
| | | | 2. Type–II | 167 |
| | | | 3. DKA | 167 |
| | | B. Liver Diseases—Jaundice | 1. Neonatal | 169 |
| | | | 2. Hemolytic | 169 |
| | | | 3. Hepatic | 170 |
| | | | 4. Obstructive | 170 |
| | | C. Acid-Base Disorders | 1. Metabolic Acidosis | 171 |
| | | | 2. Metabolic Alkalosis | 171 |
| | | | 3. Respiratory Acidosis | 172 |
| | | | 4. Respiratory Alkalosis | 172 |
| | | D. Cardiac Disease | 1. Myocardial Infarction | 173 |
| | | E. Renal Diseases | 1. Nephrotic Syndrome | 174 |
| | | | 2. Chronic Renal Failure | 174 |
| | | F. Purine Metabolism | 1. Gout | 175 |
| II. | Deficiency Disorders | A. Vitamin A | 1. Night Blindness | 176 |
| | | B. Vitamin D | 2. Rickets | 177 |
| | | C. Vitamin C | 3. Scurvy | 177 |
| | | D. Vitamin $B_{12}$ | 4. Macrocytic Anemia | 178 |
| | | E. Protein Energy Malnutrition (PEM) | 5. Kwashiorkor | 178 |
| III. | Inherited Disorders (Inborn Errors of Metabolism) | A. Carbohydrate Metabolism | 1. Lactose Intolerance | 179 |
| | | | 2. Galactosemia | 180 |
| | | | 3. Hereditary Fructose Intolerance (HFI) | 180 |
| | | B. Lipid Metabolism | 1. Familial Hypercholesterolemia (FH) | 181 |
| | | C. Amino Acid Metabolism | 1. Homocystinuria | 181 |
| | | | 2. Phenylketonuria (PKU) | 182 |
| | | | 3. Alkaptonuria | 183 |
| IV. | Hormonal Disorders | A. Thyroid Disorder | 1. Hypothyroidism | 183 |
| | | B. Parathyroid | 2. Hyerparathyroidism | 184 |

# Competency Table

| Topic: Biochemistry Laboratory Tests | | Number of competencies (22) | | Number of procedures that require certification (05) | | | Chapter/Page no. | |
| --- | --- | --- | --- | --- | --- | --- | --- | --- |
| Number | Competency The student should be able to | Core (Y/N) | Suggested teaching-learning method | Suggested assessment method | No. Required to certify | Integration: Vertical/ Horizontal | Chapter | Page no. |
| BI11.1 | Describe commonly used laboratory apparatus and equipments, good safe laboratory practice and waste disposal. | Y | Lecture, small group discussion | Written/Viva voce | | | 2 | 4 |
| BI11.2 | Describe the preparation of buffers and estimation of pH. | Y | Lecture, small group discussion | Written/Viva voce | | | 3 | 13 |
| BI11.3 | Describe the chemical components of normal urine. | Y | Lecture, small group discussion | Written/Viva voce | | | 5 | 21 |
| BI11.4 | Perform urine analysis to estimate and determine normal and abnormal constituents. | Y | DOAP session | Skill assessment | 1 | General medicine/ Physiology | 6 | 28 |
| BI11.5 | Describe the use of paper chromatography. | Y | Lecture, small group discussion | Written/Viva voce | | General medicine | 25 | 105 |
| BI11.6 | Describe the principles of colorimetry. | Y | Lecture, small group discussion | Written/Viva voce | | | 9 | 45 |
| BI11.7 | Demonstrate the estimation of serum creatinine and creatinine clearance. | Y | Practical | Skills assessment | 1 | | 13 | 62 |

*(Contd...)*

(Contd...)

| Number | Competency The student should be able to | Core (Y/N) | Suggested teaching-learning method | Suggested assessment method | No. Required to certify | Integration: Vertical/ Horizontal | Chapter | Page No. |
|---|---|---|---|---|---|---|---|---|
| BI11.8 | Demonstrate estimation of serum proteins, albumin and AG ratio. | Y | Practical | Skills assessment | 1 | | 15 | 73 |
| BI11.9 | Demonstrate estimation of serum cholesterol and HDL cholesterol. | Y | Practical | Skills assessment | | | 16 | 77 |
| BI11.10 | Demonstrate the estimation of triglycerides. | Y | Practical | Skills assessment | | | 17 | 79 |
| BI11.11 | Demonstrate estimation of calcium and phosphorous. | Y | Practical | Skills assessment | | | 18 | 82 |
| BI11.12 | Demonstrate the estimation of serum bilirubin. | Y | Practical | Skills assessment | | | 19 | 87 |
| BI11.13 | Demonstrate the estimation of SGOT/SGPT. | Y | Practical | Skills assessment | | | 20 | 90 |
| BI11.14 | Demonstrate the estimation of alkaline phosphatase. | Y | Practical | Skills assessment | | | 21 | 92 |
| BI11.15 | Describe and discuss the composition CSF. | Y | Lecture, small group discussion | Written/Viva voce | | | 8 | 41 |
| BI11.16 | Observe use of commonly used equipments/ techniques in biochemistry including:<br>• pH meter<br>• Paper chromatography of amino acid<br>• Protein electrophoresis<br>• TLC, PAGE<br>• Electrolyte analysis by ISE<br>• Autoanalyzer<br>• DNA isolation from blood/tissue | Y | Demonstration | Skill assessment | | General medicine/ Pathology | 4<br>24–33 | 16<br>103–128 |

(Contd...)

(Contd...)

| Number | Competency The student should be able to | Core (Y/N) | Suggested teaching-learning method | Suggested assessment method | No. Required to certify | Integration: Vertical/ Horizontal | Chapter | Page No. |
|---|---|---|---|---|---|---|---|---|
| BI11.17 | Explain the basis and rationale of biochemical tests done in the following conditions:<br>• Diabetes mellitus<br>• Dyslipidemia<br>• Myocardial infarction<br>• Renal failure, gout<br>• Proteinuria<br>• Nephrotic syndrome<br>• Edema<br>• Jaundice<br>• Liver diseases, pancreatitis<br>• Acid-base disorders<br>• Thyroid disorders. | Y | Lecture, small group discussion | Written/Viva voce | | | 11<br>14<br>22<br>23<br>35–40<br>43 | 51<br>68<br>94<br>101<br>137–152<br>165 |
| BI11.18 | Discuss the principles of Spectrophotometry. | Y | Lecture, small group discussion | Written/Viva voce | | | 10 | 49 |
| BI11.19 | Outline the basic principles involved in the functioning of instruments commonly used in biochemistry laboratory and their applications. | Y | Lecture, small group discussion | Written/Viva voce | | | 12<br>23–32 | 58<br>101–125 |
| BI11.20 | Identify abnormal constituents in urine, interpret the findings and correlate these with pathological states. | Y | DOAP sessions | Skill assessment | 1 | | 6<br>7 | 28<br>34 |
| BI11.21 | Demonstrate estimation of glucose, creatinine, urea and total protein in serum. | Y | DOAP sessions | Skill assessment | 1 | | 11–15 | 51–73 |

(Contd...)

(Contd...)

| Number | Competency The student should be able to | Core (Y/N) | Suggested teaching-learning method | Suggested assessment method | No. Required to certify | Integration: Vertical/ Horizontal | Chapter | Page No. |
|---|---|---|---|---|---|---|---|---|
| BI11.22 | Calculate Albumin: Globulin (AG) ratio and creatinine clearance. | Y | Lecture, small group discussion | Written/Viva voce | | General medicine | 13 15 | 62 73 |
| BI11.23 | Calculate energy content of different food items, identify food items with high and low glycemic index and explain the importance of these in the diet. | Y | Lecture, small group discussion | Written/Viva voce | | General medicine | 41 | 157 |
| BI11.24 | Enumerate advantages and/or disadvantages of use of unsaturated, saturated and trans fats in food. | Y | Lecture, small group discussion | Written/Viva voce | | General medicine | 42 | 160 |
| PY4.8 | Describe and discuss gastric function tests, pancreatic exocrine tests and liver function tests. | Y | Lecture, small group discussion | Written/Viva voce | | | 34–36 | 133–144 |
| PY7.8 | Describe and discuss renal function tests. | Y | Lecture, small group discussion | Written/Viva voce | | | 38 | 145 |
| PY8.4 | Describe function tests: Thyroid gland, adrenal cortex, adrenal medulla and pancreas | Y | Lecture, small group discussion | Written/Viva voce | | | 39 40 | 148 152 |

DOAP session—Demonstrate, Observe, Assess, Perform

# Plate 1

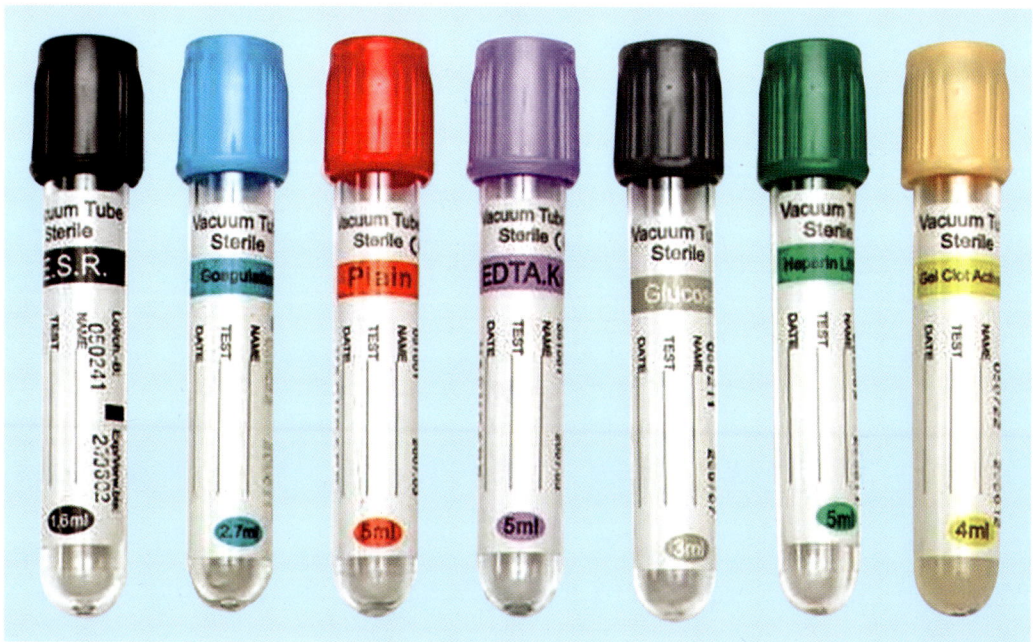

**Page 8:** Vacutainer.

# SECTION 1

# General

## Section Outline

1. General Instructions
2. Laboratory Equipments and Procedures
   A. Commonly used laboratory equipments
   B. Good safe laboratory procedures and safety rules
   C. Laboratory waste disposal
   D. Collection and handling of samples
3. Buffers and pH
4. Quality Control

# CHAPTER 1

# General Instructions

## ■ BIOCHEMISTRY PRACTICALS: GENERAL INSTRUCTIONS TO THE STUDENTS

1. All the students should be punctual in attending practical classes. All should wear neat white coat. Dresses made by inflammable materials should be avoided.
2. All should attend the instruction or demonstration classes before each practical class.
3. Students can leave the laboratory only after finishing their practicals and getting signature in the observation book.
4. All the glasswares should be cleaned thoroughly and all waste materials should be dropped into the waste basket.
5. After using, all the reagent bottles should be closed with stoppers and kept in the appropriate places in the racks.
6. While taking the bottles from the rack, students should hold the bottles with both hands. Should not carry the bottles by the neck.
7. Pipetting by mouth should be avoided. Students can use teats whenever necessary. Should not pipette concentrated acids, alkali or toxic chemicals by mouth.
8. All burners should be put off after the practical work is over.
9. In the event of any accident such as spilling of acid or alkali over the body or eye, accidental entry of acid/alkali into the mouth during pipetting, electric shock, gas leakage, burns etc. It should be informed immediately to the staff for first aid and emergency treatments.
10. All the students should maintain a Biochemistry record notebook prescribed by the college and submit them within the stipulated time. Separate marks are allotted for records as per the instruction of the University.
11. Every student should maintain an 'Assessment Record' individually—for recording the scores/grades for the Formative Assessments for each and every sessions performed by them and also for Certification of Skills

# CHAPTER 2

# Laboratory Equipments and Procedures

**BI11.1** Describe commonly used laboratory apparatus and equipment, good safe laboratory practice and waste disposal.

## A. COMMONLY USED LABORATORY EQUIPMENTS

1. **Weighing balances**: Different types of balances are used to weigh even minute amount of reagents and chemicals.
   a. Double pan chemical balance.

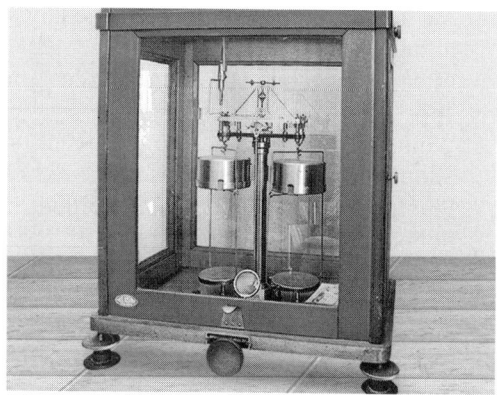

   b. Single pan electric/electronic balances.

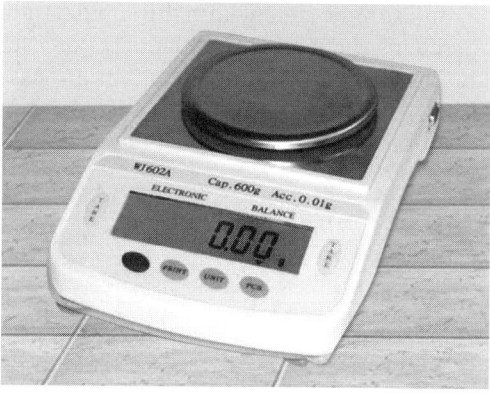

## Chapter 2: Laboratory Equipments and Procedures

2. **Centrifuges:** Used to separate sediment particles in a liquid suspension by means of centrifugal force under different speed with the help of electric motor. Four or Eight test tubes (buckets) can be used.
   Types of centrifuges are:
   a. Table top model
   b. Cold centrifuge
   c. Ultra centrifuge: Used to separate cellular sediments.

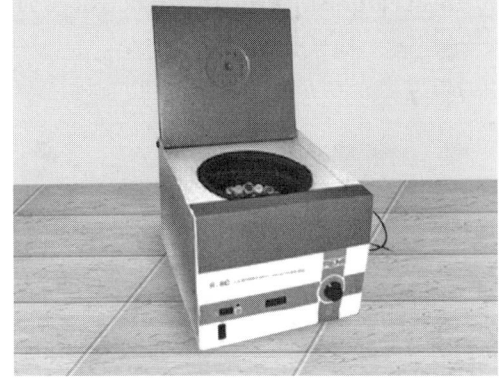

3. **Water bath:** Electrically heated water baths in which temperature can be controlled and regulated. Boiling water bath has temperature control of 100°C.

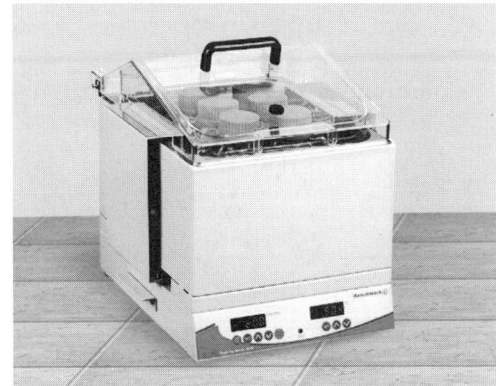

4. **Hot air oven:** It has temperature ranges upto 250°C. It is used for drying and sterilizing glasswares.
5. **Incubator:** Used to regulate temperature thermostatically. Mainly used in enzyme estimations using buffers at a particular temperature.

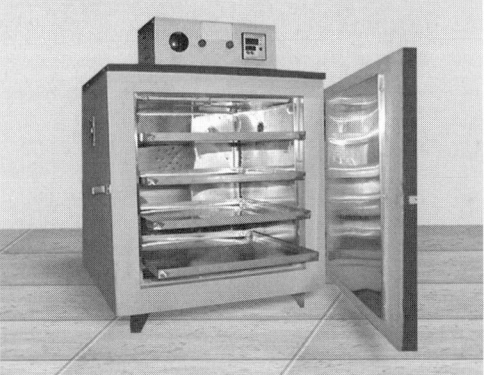

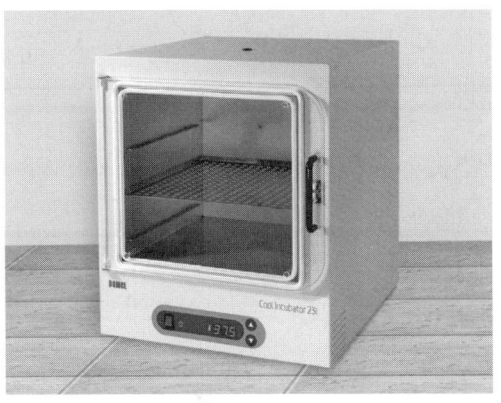

6. **Desiccators:** Used to dry or keep dry solid or liquid substances.

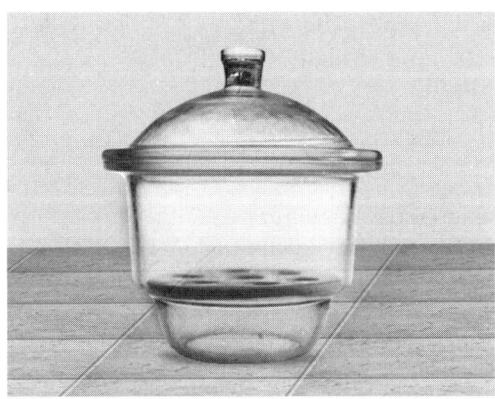

7. **Commonly used glassware items:**

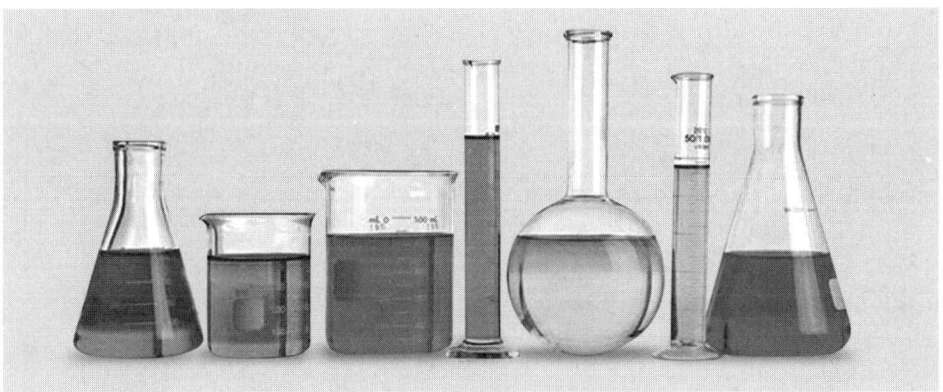

   a. *Test tubes*: Various sizes—5 mL to 30 mL; graduated or non-graduated. Serum tubes are used to collect samples or to centrifuge.

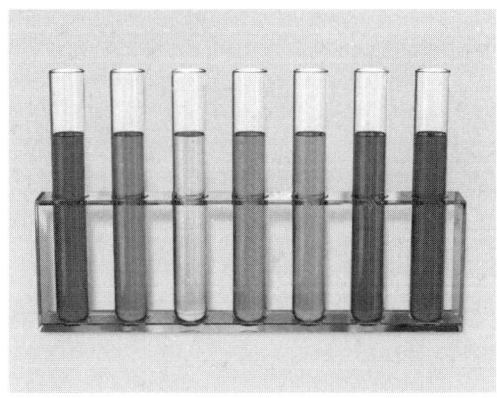

b. *Conical flasks*: Used for heating solutions and for titrations.

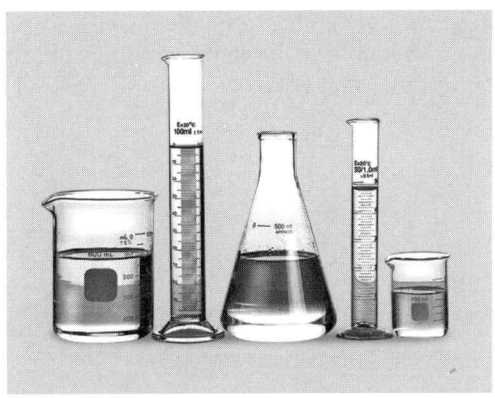

c. *Volumetric flasks*: Used for preparing standard solutions. Fixed volume flasks.

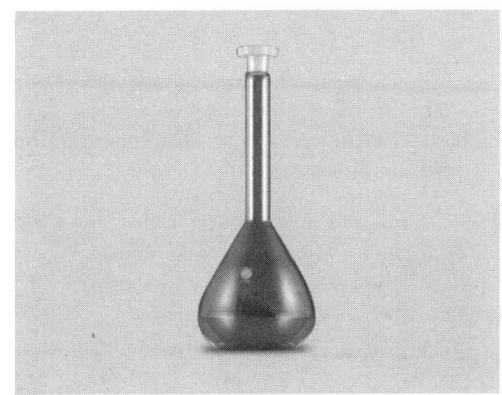

d. *Measuring cylinders*: Graduated and in different sizes are available (10 mL to 2 L). Used for reagent preparations.
e. *Beakers*: Available in different sizes—in glass or in plastic. Used to prepare reagent and to store.
f. *Pipettes*: Available from 0.1 mL to 25 mL volume. Graduated pipettes: Used to deliver accurate quantity of liquid. They are of two types—Blowout and Non-blowout varieties.

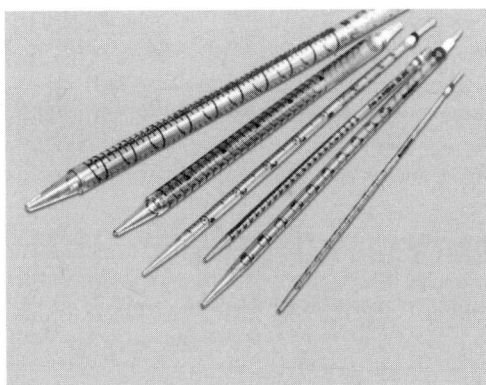
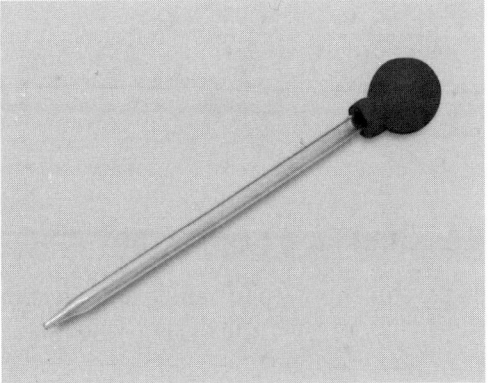

g. *Automated micropipettes:*
Used to transfer micro-volumes of samples: 1 microliter (μL), 10 μL, 50 μL, 100 μL, etc.
1 μL = 0.001 mL.

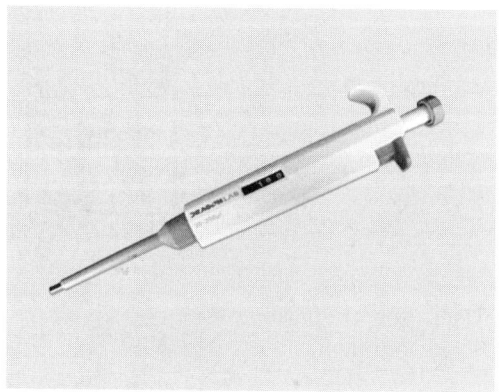

h. *Vacutainer:* They are sample collection tubes with specific color codes as per the nature of the blood samples as noted in the picture given below.

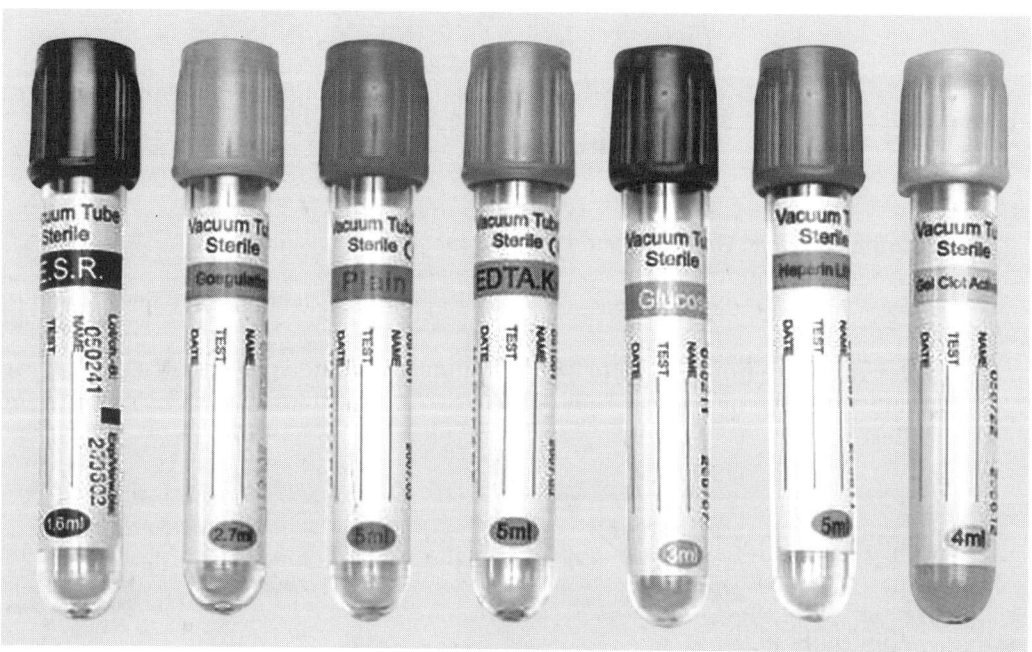

## ■ B. GOOD SAFE LABORATORY PROCEDURES AND SAFETY RULES

As the students have to handle lots chemicals, glasswares and biological samples everybody should be very careful in dealing with them.

## Precautions to be Taken

- Overcoats and gloves should be worn.
- Should not eat or drink anything inside the laboratory.
- Hand washings should be done regularly before and after the lab work.
- Should not carry the reagent bottles by neck. Should use both hands to carry the bottles.
- Inflammable reagents should be kept away from fire.
- Mouth pipetting should be avoided always. Teats can be used.
- Hair should be tied up.

## Good Housekeeping

- Availability of first aid box
- Availability of fire extinguishers
- Labeling of all chemicals and proper storage
- Work area: Should be clean and all waste items should be discarded in the dustbin then and there.
- Sterilization should be done using non-inflammable disinfectants
- All needles and syringes should be destroyed immediately
- All electrical equipments should be connected with safety measures and earthed properly.

## First Aid Measures

- **Acid burns—Over skin:** Should be washed under running water and after drying should be soaked in 5% aqueous sodium carbonate solution.
- **Chemical injury to the eyes:** Washing with water and the corner of the eyes should be rinsed. The student should be then referred to the ophthalmologist.
- **Accidental swallowing of acid:** Mouth should be washed with water and to drink water followed by milk in acid swallowing and lime juice in case of alkali swallowing.
- **Inhalation injury:** The person should be taken to a well aerated area without contamination and should be given hot water or warm drink.
- **Cut injury:** Wound should be washed under running water. Any glass pieces if present should be removed and bleeding to be stopped by using tight bandage or compression. The patient should be then taken to the casualty for further treatment.
- **First aid box:** Should be available which should contain the following:
  - Sterilized Gauze and cotton
  - Sterilized eye pads
  - Wash bottle—for eye washing
  - Bandage materials
  - Emergency injections—Adrenaline, Steroids, etc.
  - Adhesive plaster
  - Scissors
  - Antiseptic lotion.

## ■ C. LABORATORY WASTE DISPOSAL

- To avoid the risk of biological hazards all the wastes and infected materials should be disposed safely. All the chemical wastes, left over samples, gloves, needles and containers should be disposed with due care.

**Section 1:** General

- All the wastes should be segregated and disposed in color coded bags—Yellow, Red, White and Blue bags.

## Type I—Biomedical Wastes

| Category | Type of Waste |
|---|---|
| Yellow Bags | - Cotton swabs<br>- Leftover samples<br>- Placenta, postoperative body wastes<br>- Anatomical/Pathological wastes<br>- Dressing material<br>- Contaminated samples with blood and other samples<br>- Discarded drugs<br>- Discarded linen, beddings |
| Red Bags | - Syringes without needles<br>- IV sets<br>- Catheters<br>- Gloves<br>- Urine bags<br>- IV bottles<br>- Vacutainers |
| White (Translucent) Bags | - Needles<br>- Syringes with fixed needles<br>- Blades<br>- Scalpels<br>- Contaminated metal sharps |
| Blue Bags | - Needles:<br>  – Broken glass<br>  – Ampoules<br>  – Lab slides<br>- Metals:<br>  – Nails<br>  – Metallic body implants<br>  – Scissors |

- Other sharp items should be soaked in 1% bleaching powder solution and then separated in cardboard boxes
- Items soiled with blood should be soakd in 1% sodium hypochlorite solution and washed or packed in yellow bags for incineration.

## Type II—General Wastes

All the wastes other than biomedical waste which has not been in contact with any hazardous, chemical or biological secretions are included in this group. It consists of:
1. Newspapers, paper and cardboard boxes
2. Plastic water bottles
3. Aluminum cans of soft drink
4. Packaging materials

5. Food containers after emptying the food
6. Organic or biodegradable waste—food waste
7. Construction and demolition wastes.

They can be disposed in black bags as per solid waste management rules.

## ■ D. COLLECTION AND HANDLING OF SAMPLES

Analysis of various parameters in different types of samples is being done in the biochemical laboratories to diagnose many diseases routinely. Collection of the samples should be done at a common collection center after verifying the name, age, sex, address and ID of the patient and entering it in the concerned register and the date and time of collection should also be noted.

## Types of Samples

- Blood
- Urine
- CSF
- Ascitic fluid
- Pleural fluid
- Pericardial fluid
- Saliva
- Sweat
- Gastric secretions
- Calculi

Blood and urine are the commonly used specimens for investigations.

## Collection of Blood

Blood can be collected from veins, arteries or capillaries. Usually venous blood is preferable. Arterial blood is mainly taken for analyzing blood gas. Clean and dry empty containers (small bottles or serum tubes) are used. It should be labeled properly. Under strict aseptic precautions, venous blood should be collected usually from the cubital veins or from the veins of the dorsum of hands. For infants and small children, blood can be collected from femoral veins.

To avoid hemolysis of blood, the following precautions should be taken:
1. The container should be clean and dry.
2. Syringe and needle should be sterile and dry.
3. Blood should be withdrawn gently and gentle pressure should be given to the piston to transfer the blood to the container.
4. After collection, the specimen should be kept aside. No shaking should be done.
Hemolyzed blood will alter the values of many parameters.

### *Components of Blood*

1. **Plasma** is the supernatant got after centrifuging the blood which contains an anticoagulant. It differs from serum by having fibrinogen.
2. **Serum** is the straw colored fluid obtained from the normal blood after coagulation. It does not contain fibrinogen.

Anticoagulants and preservatives used for obtaining plasma:
1. **Heparin-mucopolysaccharide (costly):** Used mostly 2 mg/10 mL blood
2. **Ethylene diamine tetra-acetate (EDTA):**
   - Chelating agent
   - Used for hematological examinations. 15–150 mg/10 mL blood

3. **Sodium fluoride:** Preservative and anticoagulant for blood glucose. It inhibits the enzyme Enolase and stops further degradation of glucose to pyruvate.
4. **Oxalates:** Inhibits by forming soluble complexes with calcium ions (>3 mg/mL-hemolysis) Potassium oxalate 1–2 mg/mL of blood.
5. **Citrate (for hematocrits):** 30–60 mg/10 mL of blood
6. **Iodoacetate:** Substitute for sodium fluoride.

## Collection of Urine

One time specimen-usually early morning midstream specimen is used for qualitative analysis. 24 hours urine should be collected from 6 AM to the next day 6 AM for estimating important biochemical parameters.

### Preservatives for Collection of 24 hours Urine

Formalin, thymol, chloroform, toluene, concentrated hydrochloric acid, glacial acetic acid.

# CHAPTER 3

# Buffers and pH

**BI11.2** Describe the preparation of buffers and estimation of pH.

## ■ PREPARATION OF BUFFERS AND ESTIMATION OF pH

**Buffers:** They are a mixture of weak acid and its salts with strong base or a mixture of weak base and its salt with strong acid. When a small amount of acid or base is added, a buffer can resist the change in pH.

**Acids:** They are proton donors and bases are proton acceptors. When a strong acid is added to a buffer the H⁺ ions donated by the acid are accepted by the base member A⁻ of the buffer to get its acid member (HA). In contrast rise in OH ions is neutralised by the proton donated by the acid number (HA) with the formation of conjugate base (A⁻).

## Dissociation Constant (Ka)

The dissociation of an acid is a freely reversible reaction. At equilibrium the ratio between the dissociated and undissociated particles is a constant.

$$Ka = \frac{[H^+][A^-]}{[HA]}$$

The pH at which the acid is half ionized is called pKa of an acid which is a constant at a particular temperature and pressure

$$pH = -\log[H^+] = \frac{\log 1}{[H^+]}$$

pH is defined as the negative logarithm of the hydrogen ion concentration. $pH = -\log(H)^+$

**Buffer capacity:** It is the gram equivalent of acid or alkali required by one liter of a buffer to undergo a charge of pH by 1. A buffer which requires more acid or alkali is said to have more buffer capacity.

## Preparation of Buffers

**Phosphate Buffer:** (pH 5.8–7.4)
- 35.61 g of disodium monophosphate is dissolved in water and the volume is adjusted to 1000 mL to prepare: Solution A (0.2 M)

- 27.6 g of monosodium dihydrogen phosphate is dissolved separately in water and this volume is also adjusted to 1000 mL to prepare: Solution B (0.2 M)
- Solution A and B are mixed and the pH is adjusted by using either acid (phosphoric acid) or alkali sodium hydroxide.
- **Example:**
  - To get a solution with pH 7.4, 19 mL of Solution A: Disodium monohydrogen phosphate and 81 mL of Solution B: Monosodium dihydrogen phosphate are mixed
  - By using this principle, Acetate buffer and Tris: HCl buffer can be prepared.

## Estimation of pH

pH is defined as the negative logarithm of the hydrogen ion concentration.

### pH = – log (H)⁺

pH values of some important biological fluids.
- Blood: 7.4
- Bile: 7.6 Alkaline
- Pancreatic Juice: 8.8
- Saliva, Human milk: 6.7
- Urine: 6.0 Acidic
- Gastric Juice: 1.77

## Determination of pH

### By Using Indicators

Indicators are substances which change their color with variation of pH of the solution. Examples of indicators are:
- **Thymol blue:** pH 1.2–2.8
- **Methyl red:** pH 4.3–6.1 (Red in acid medium, yellow in alkaline medium)
- **Phenol red:** pH range of 6.8–8.4. It is red in alkaline and yellow in acid medium.
- **Phenolphthalein:** pH range of 8.3–10.0.
  It is used as an indicator for titration of total acidity of gastric juice. End point is faint pink color.

### By Using pH Paper

- **Litmus paper:** Red in acid, Blue in alkali.
- **Indicator:** Standard colors with pH range, will be compared with the paper dipped in test solution.

  A strip of indicator paper is moistened in the given solution and the color produced is compared to the color chart to know the pH.

### By Using pH Meter (Fig. 3.1)

This apparatus is used to determine the pH of a solution more accurately by potential measurement of certain electrodes.

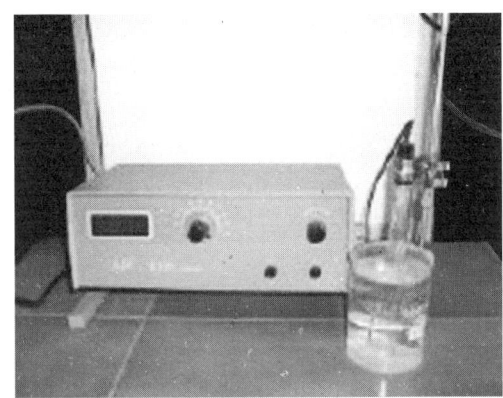

Fig. 3.1: pH meter.

## Electrometric Determination of pH

**Principle:** When a glass membrane separates two different solutions having different pH, a potential difference is found to be present between the surfaces of the glass. The potential is measured against a standard calomel electrode.

### Parts of a pH Meter

1. Potentiometer.
2. **Reference calomel electrode:** It has metallic mercury in contact with mercuric chloride in potassium chloride solution.
3. **Glass electrode:** It is a bulb of special glass which is filled with some standard electrolytes such as O.I.N HCl in contact with a suitable metallic electrode.
4. Solution of Known pH.

### Operation of pH Meter

pH meter is turned 15 minutes prior to use and then it is calibrated with reference buffers. Then the electrodes are dipped in the test solution for 30 seconds and the reading is taken. The glass electrodes should be carefully washed after each pH determination.

# CHAPTER 4

# Quality Control

**BI11.16** Observe use of commonly used equipment/techniques in biochemistry **including concepts of Quality Control.**

## ■ QUALITY CONTROL

Quality control (QC) is an integral part of the regular and accurate function of a clinical chemistry laboratory. Quality confirms the reliability of each test performed on a sample to satisfy the expectations of the patients. Corrective measures are taken promptly if there are errors which may be due to pre- and postanalytical variables.

This QC program can be implemented in two ways: Internal and External quality control.
1. **Internal QC:** This type of checking is done once or twice in a month. Here the routine laboratory tests are assessed and evaluated on a daily basis. The peripheral laboratory prepares a reference standard sample and checks the results on the daily basis. This is called the Internal Quality Control.
2. **External QC:** In this type, a central reference laboratory sends a serum sample of known concentration to the peripheral smaller laboratory. The sample is analyzed there and if the results are the same or close to the correct report, the procedures followed in the peripheral laboratory are reliable. There will be a tie up of smaller laboratories with reference laboratories to conduct this program. This can be repeated at regular intervals—once or twice a month.
   - *Accuracy*: It is the measure of closeness of the estimated value to the true value. If two technicians X and Y-perform the analysis of a sample containing 28 mg/dL of urea, and if the result obtained by the technician X is 22 mg/dL and that of the technician Y is 26 mg/dL, the result of the technician Y is more accurate than that of technician X. This is known as the accuracy of the result.
   - *Precision*: Precision depends on the technique, the reagents used and also the technical ability of the technician. Precision is the measure of the reproducibility of the result. If a technician performs blood urea estimation on the same sample on three or four occasions and the results obtained will be 22 mg/dL, 24 mg/dL, and 28 mg/dL, the results are reproduces well and the precision is good.
   - *Specificity*: It is determined by the method of analysis. Specificity means that one substance should answer a particular test. For the estimation of glucose, glucose oxidase

method is specific to glucose only and it will not analyse other reducing sugars such as galactose etc.
- *Sensitivity*: It denotes whether a method is capable of measuring a particular substance in a very low concentration or in dilute solution. For example, a few grams of protein in serum is estimated by Biuret method whereas by Spectrophotometer few milligrams of proteins can be estimated. On the other hand, by ELISA method we can measure even a microgram of protein/dL. So ELISA method is the most sensitive method.

A test should be both sensitive and sensitive. When the sensitivity is increased, the specificity is decreased.

## Total Quality Management (TQM)

- Six sigma principles and metrics were introduced in laboratory testing processes.
- Five Qs in quality management are: Quality planning, Quality laboratory process, Quality control, Quality assurance and Quality improvement.
- There should be commitment, resources and technical competence to implement good quality assurance in the laboratory.
- Quality control refers to technical procedures used in quality assurance programmes – which include control of preanalytical variables, analytical variables and the quality of analysis.

### *Quality Control Charts*

- They are used to compare the control values with the control limits. It provides a visual display for quick review.
- Daily QC chart should be available in the laboratory.
- The control chart helps to detect accuracy problems (Shift in mean) and precision problem (shift in SD)
- There may be inherent random error which are denoted by graphs plotted using error on the y-axis and probability on the x-axis.

### *Levy Jenning's Chart (LJ)*

During each run the control specimen are analysed and the value plotted on the chart. When the control values are within the control limits patient's values can be reported. Reporting should be stopped even if a single control value is out of limit. After the problem is resolved the run is repeated.

### *Westgard's Multirule Chart*

Here the same LJ chart procedures are done using two different controls.

### *External Quality Assessment Schemes (EQAS)*

- This compares the performance of different laboratories
- It maintains long-term accuracy of analytical methods
- The summary of reports are sent to the participating laboratories
- For each analyte the standard deviation index (SDI) is calculated by using the student "t" test
- When the difference is significant from a particular laboratory, that laboratory is cautioned
- SDI = Lab result – Group mean/Groups SD.

# SECTION 2

# Analysis of Urine and Cerebrospinal Fluid

## Section Outline

5. Normal Urine: Characteristics and Analysis
6. Abnormal Constituents of Urine
7. Screening of Urine for Inborn Errors of Metabolism and the Use of Paper Chromatography
8. Composition of Cerebrospinal Fluid

# CHAPTER 5
# Normal Urine: Characteristics and Analysis

**BI11.3** Describe the chemical components of normal urine.

## ■ NORMAL URINE

Urine is an excretory product of the body produced by the kidneys. Examination of urine may lead to the diagnosis of many metabolic and systemic diseases.

## ■ SPECIMEN COLLECTION

1. Fresh midstream specimen of 10–20 mL is collected in a clean dry container.
2. 24 hours urine collection-for total urinary proteins, calcium, certain hormonal assays. This requires addition of preservatives such as 2N hydrochloric acid, conc. sulfuric acid, crystals of thymol or 10% acetic acid, etc. depending upon the type of tests. Routine urinary examination may be carried out under the following three headings:
   i. Physical examination
   ii. Chemical examination
   iii. Microscopic examination (not needed).

## ■ PHYSICAL CHARACTERISTICS

### 1. Appearance

a. Freshly voided normal urine is clear and transparent.
   On standing it may become turbid due to the bacterial action that converts urea to ammonium carbonate. This makes urine alkaline and causes precipitation of phosphates or oxalates or urates.
b. Abnormal urine may be turbid due to:
   1. Presence of pus cells in urinary tract infections (UTI)
   2. Increased excretion of phosphates in alkaline urine.
   3. Chyluria (milky white urine) presence of fat globules due to obstruction in the lymphatics of urinary tract as in filariasis.

### 2. Color

a. **Normal urine:** Straw or amber-yellow in color due to the presence of the pigment Urochrome. Concentrated urine will be dark yellow in color due to low water intake. Yellow colored urine will be present in people who consume vitamin B complex. Certain food items also will change the color of normal urine.

b. **Abnormal urine:**
   1. Deep yellow: Jaundiced due to the presence of bile pigments.
   2. Reddish: Hematuria—due to stones in the urinary tract, carcinoma of urinary bladder, injury to the urinary passage, stricture of the urethra.
   3. Reddish brown: Hemoglobinuria—incompatible blood transfusion.
   4. Milky white: Chyluria—filariasis.
   5. Black on standing: Alkaptonuria—due to the presence of homogentisic acid (inborn error of metabolism of tyrosine).

## 3. Volume

a. **Normal urine:** 800–2000 mL/day. Day output is greater than night output.
   *Factors influencing volume are:*
   1. Quantity of fluids intake
   2. Quality of food taken
   3. Climate—output is low in hot climate due to excessive sweating
   4. Physical exercise.
b. **Abnormal urine:**
   1. *Polyuria:* Increased volume—due to:
      a. Diabetes mellitus
      b. Diabetes insipidus
      c. Later stages of chronic renal failure
      d. Drugs: Diuretics.
   2. *Oliguria:* Decreased volume (less than 500 mL)—due to:
      a. Excess of fluid loss due to vomiting, diarrhea
      b. Acute nephritis.
   3. *Anuria:* Total absence of urine—due to:
      a. Shock
      b. Acute tubular necrosis
      c. Blood transfusion reaction
      d. Bilateral renal stones.

   The ratio of day urine to night urine is 2:1 or 3:1. The ratio may be altered in renal diseases.

## 4. Odor

- *Normal*: Fresh urine—aromatic odor.
- *Abnormal odor*
    - Putrid or ammoniacal odor: Bacterial decomposition
    - Fruity odor: Diabetic ketoacidosis
    - Mousy odor: Phenylketonuria.

## 5. Specific Gravity

- *Normal urine*: 1.015–1.025
- *High specific gravity*

- Restricted water intake
- Presence of glucose in urine (diabetes mellitus)
- Presence of albumin in urine (albuminuria)

*Low specific gravity*:
- Polyuria (except diabetes mellitus)
- High fluid intake
- Diabetes insipidus.

Specific gravity is measured with urinometer. Specific gravity is directly proportionate to the concentration of solutes excreted.

## CHEMICAL CHARACTERISTICS

## 1. Acidity/pH

The pH of normal urine is 4.6–8 (average 6). Freshly voided urine is acidic. On standing it may become alkaline due to the formation of ammonia from bacterial decomposition. pH of urine is influenced by the nature of diet.

**High protein diet or low carbohydrate diet:** Acidic urine.
**Vegetables and fruits:** Alkaline urine.

## 2. Constituents of Normal Urine

- **Inorganic constituents:** Chloride, calcium, phosphorus, inorganic sulfates, ammonia, sodium, potassium, magnesium.
- **Organic constituents:** Urea, uric acid, creatine, creatinine, ethereal sulfate (Also urobilinogen, hippuric acid, indican).

### A. Inorganic Constituents

1. **Chloride ($Cl^-$)** Chief anion in urine
   - Normal: 10–12 g of chloride as NaCl/day.
   
   **Decreased urinary chloride**
   - Excessive sweating
   - Fasting
   - Diarrhea and vomiting
   - Diabetes insipidus
   - Cushing's syndrome
   - Infections
   
   **Increased urinary chloride**
   - Excessive intake of fluids
   - Addison's disease

2. **Calcium:** Normal excretion—0.1–0.3 g/day
   High level: Hyperparathyroidism
              : Hyperthyroidism
              : Hypervitaminosis D
              : Multiple myeloma.

3. **Phosphates**
   *Normal value*: 0.8–1.3 g/day.
   (Presenting as inorganic as well as organic phosphates.)
   *Increased in*: Bone diseases—Rickets, osteomalacia, parathyroid dysfunction.
   *Decreased in*: Diarrhea
   - Infections
   - Nephritis
   - Hypoparathyroidism
   - Pregnancy.
4. **Ammonia:** (Normal excretion 0.7 g/day). Excreted as ammonium salts.
   Increased in acidosis. Decreased in alkalosis.
5. **Sulfates**
   Three forms of sulfates:
   i. Inorganic sulfates (of Na and K) 80–85%
   ii. Organic sulfates—ethereal sulfates 5%
   iii. Neutral sulfur (organic sulphates) 15–20%.
   They are derived from the metabolism of sulfur containing amino acids such as cysteine, cystine and methionine.
   *Normal value of total inorganic sulfates*: 0.7–1 g/day
   *Increased in*: High protein diet
   *Decreased in*: Renal dysfunction.

## B. Organic Constituents

1. **Ethereal sulfates (Organic) (5%)**
   **Normal value:** 0.06–0.12 g/day. It consists of Na and K salts of sulfuric acid, esters of phenols such as indoxyl etc. They are formed during putrefaction of amino acids in the intestines.
   Urinary sulfates: Increased in:
   - *Inherited disorders*: Cystinuria, homocystinuria.
   - *Cyanide poisoning*: Thiocyanate.
2. **Urea**
   Major nitrogenous constituent of urine. It is produced from the breakdown of proteins.
   *Normal urinary urea*: 15–30 g/24 hours.
   *Increased in*:
   - (Increased protein catabolism)
   - High protein diet.
   - Fever
   - Diabetes mellitus.
   *Decreased in:*
   - Low protein diet
   - Liver diseases
   - Nephritis
   - Acidosis.
3. **Uric acid**
   It is the end product of purine catabolism in humans.
   *Normal value*: 0.5–1 g/day.
   *Increased in*: Leukemias especially during cytotoxic drug therapy.

- Wilson's disease.
- Administration of cortisone/ACTH.

4. **Creatinine**
   It is the anhydride of creatine. Urinary creatinine is derived from muscle creatine. It is not influenced by the protein intake. Normal Value 1–2 g/24 hrs.
   *Increased in*: Fever, myopathy.

5. **Urobilinogen**
   Normal urine contains traces of urobilinogen, which is derived from bilirubin by the action of bacterial flora in the intestine, enters into circulation and then excreted by the kidneys.
   Increased urobilinogen: Hemolytic jaundice, liver diseases.
   Absence of urobilinogen: Obstructive jaundice.

## Composition of Normal Urine

- **Solids:** 60 g/L
- **Water:** 1200 mL.

# ANALYSIS OF NORMAL URINE

(Each student can collect his/her urine in a 100 mL beaker and perform the following tests)

| Experiment | Observation | Inference |
|---|---|---|
| **I. Physical Examination** | | |
| 1. Color | Straw colored | Due to the presence of urochrome |
| 2. Appearance | Clear | Normal urine is clear and transparent |
| 3. Reaction (pH) test the pH by using pH paper or litmus paper | pH of the given urine is—(acidic or alkaline) | pH of normal urine is 4.6–8.0 (average 6.0) |
| 4. Specific gravity test: Fill 3/4 of glass cylinder with urine. Float the urinometer without touching the sides. Note the mark on the stem of the urinometer coinciding to the surface of urine. That gives the specific gravity of urine. | Specific gravity of the given urine is— | Normal specific gravity of urine is 1.015–1.025 |
| **II. Chemical Reactions** | | |
| **A. Inorganic Constituents** | | |
| **1. Test for Chloride** To 3 mL of urine taken in a test tube, 0.5 mL of conc. nitric acid is added and mixed. 1 mL of 3% silver nitrate solution is then added. | A white precipitate of silver chloride is formed | Shows the presence of chlorides |
| **2. Test for Calcium and Phosphorus** To 10 mL of urine, 5–10 drops of strong ammonia is added and boiled, and cooled. After 5 minutes, a white precipitate is formed. Filter it and discard the filtrate. Add 5 mL of dilute acetic acid through the sides of the filter paper. Pierce the filter paper with a glass rod. Collect this in a test tube and divide it into two parts: | | |

*(Contd...)*

(Contd...)

| Experiment | Observation | Inference |
|---|---|---|
| i. To one part add 2 mL of 2% potassium oxalate solution | A white precipitate is obtained (calcium oxalate). | It shows the presence of calcium in urine. |
| ii. To the 2nd part add 1 mL of conc. $HNO_3$ and 3 mL of ammonium molybdate | A canary yellow precipitate is obtained (ammonium phosphomolybdate). | Indicates the presence of phosphorus in urine. |
| **3. Test for Ammonia** <br> To 2 mL of urine add a drop of phenolphthalein indicator. Mix and add 2% sodium carbonate drop by drop with constant mixing till a pink color is got. Boil this solution. While boiling, keep a glass rod dipped in phenolphthalein indicator near the mouth of the tube. | Phenolphthalein indicator in the glass rod changes to pink color. | The appearance of pink color is due to evolution of ammonia from decomposition of ammonia salts in urine. |
| **4. Test for Inorganic Sulfates** <br> Take 5 mL of urine in a test tube. Add 1 mL of conc. hydrochloric acid. Mix well and add 5 mL of 10% barium chloride. | A white precipitate of barium sulphate is formed. | This indicates the presence of inorganic sulfates in urine. |
| **B. Organic Constituents** | | |
| **1. Test for Ethereal Sulfates** <br> Filter off the precipitate got in above experiment. Boil the filtrate. | A white precipitate of barium sulfate is obtained. | The filtrate from the above experiment already contains excess $BaCl_2$ and HCl. Free sulfate is formed from organic sulfate by heating with HCl which reacts with barium chloride to form a white precipitate of barium sulfate. |
| **2. Test for Urea** <br> **a. Alkaline Hypobromite Test** <br> To 3 mL of urine, 5 drops of freshly prepared alkaline hypobromite solution is added and mixed. | Brisk effervescence is produced. | Shows the presence of urea in urine. |
| **b. Specific Urease Test** <br> To 3 mL of urine, 3 drops of phenolphthalein indicator is added and mixed. Then a spatulaful of horsegram powder containing urease is added and mixed and the tube is rolled between the palms. | A pink color develops. | Presence of urea is confirmed. |
| **3. Test for Uric acid** <br> **a. Benedict's Uric Acid Test** <br> To 3 mL of urine, 1 mL of phosphotungstic acid (Benedict's uric acid reagent) and 1 mL of 20% sodium carbonate solution are added and mixed. | A deep blue color is formed. | Shows the presence of uric acid in urine. |

(Contd...)

(Contd...)

| Experiment | Observation | Inference |
|---|---|---|
| **b. Schiff's Test**<br>A piece of filter paper is moistened with few drops of ammoniacal silver nitrate solution and then 2–3 drops of urine is added on the same paper. | A black color develops. | Confirms the presence of uric acid which reduces silver nitrate to metallic silver. |
| **4. Test for Creatinine (Jaffe's Test)**<br>3 mL of urine and 3 mL of water are taken in 2 separate test tubes. 1 mL of saturated picric acid and 10 drops of 10% sodium hydroxide are added to both the test tubes and mixed. Wait for 5 minutes. | A deep orange color is developed in the test tube containing urine and yellow color in the test tube containing water. | Orange color indicates the presence of creatinine in urine. |
| **5. Test for Urobilinogen**<br>To 5 mL of voided urine 1 mL of Ehrlich reagent (p-dimethylaminobenzaldehyde) is added. | A red color is seen when viewed through the mouth of the test tube. | Urobilinogen reacts with p-dimethylaminobenzaldehyde of the reagent to give red color. On standing, urobilinogen is oxidized to urobilin which does not answer this test. |

**Result:** The reactions of the constituents of normal urine are thus studied.

# CHAPTER 6

# Abnormal Constituents of Urine

**BI11.4** Perform urine analysis to estimate and determine normal and abnormal constituents.
**BI11.20** Identify abnormal constituents in urine, interpret the findings and correlate these with pathological states.

## ABNORMAL CHEMICAL CONSTITUENTS OF URINE

In diseased conditions urine may contain certain abnormal constituents. Presence of these constituents in urine will help in the diagnosis of diseased conditions.

They may be:

## 1. Reducing Sugars (Mainly Glucose)—Glycosuria

| | |
|---|---|
| Glucose: | Diabetes mellitus, Renal glycosuria. |
| Fructose: | Disorders of fructose metabolism |
| | Essential fructosuria |
| | Hereditary fructose intolerance. |
| Galactose: | Galactosemia |
| Lactose: | Pregnancy, lactating woman. |
| Pentose: | Disorder of uronic acid pathway (Essential pentosuria) |

Non-sugars such as homogentisic acid (Alkaptonuria), vitamin C and some glucuronates will also give a positive result for Benedict's test.

### Test for Reducing Sugar—Benedict's Test

To 5 mL of Benedict's reagent, 8 drops of urine is added and boiled and allowed to cool. Green or yellow or red precipitate is obtained depending upon the amount of reducing sugar present in it.

Color of the precipitate indicates the amount of glucose present in the urine of Diabetes mellitus cases.

Light green turbidity: 0.1–0.5%   Green precipitate: 0.5–1%
Yellow precipitate: 1–2%   Red precipitate: >2%

## 2. Proteins (Mainly Albumin)—Albuminuria

The amount of protein excreted normally in 24 hours urine is insignificant and it is less than 20–80 mg per day. When proteins appear in detectable quantities in urine, it is called proteinuria (albuminuria). Normal glomeruli of kidneys do not permit molecules with mol. wt more than 60,000 to pass through. But when the glomeruli are damaged, they become more permeable and allow the leakage of proteins which will be present in urine. As albumin has got smaller molecular weight it passes through the glomeruli more easily. Bence Jones proteins will be present in urine in multiple myeloma.

## Types of Proteinuria and their Causes

a. Functional proteinuria : Long Standing
: Violent Exercise
: Cold bathing
: Pregnancy

b. Organic proteinuria
   i. Prerenal : Cardiac diseases
: Abdominal tumors
: Cancer
: Collagen diseases
: Fevers, anemia, etc.
   ii. Renal : Acute and chronic glomerulonephritis
: TB kidneys
: Nephrotic syndrome.
   iii. Postrenal : (False proteinuria)
: Proteins do not pass through kidneys
: Inflammatory conditions of kidney, ureter, bladder, prostate, etc.
: Bleeding in genitourinary tract.

## Tests for Proteins

### a. Heat coagulation test

3/4 of the test tube is filled with urine and the top portion of the tube is heated by holding the tube at the bottom. A turbidity is seen on the heated portion only. 2 drops of 1% acetic acid is added. A cloudy white precipitate is seen at the top portion. Acetic acid is added to dissolve the phosphates.

### b. Sulfosalicylic acid test

To 2 mL of urine, few drops of 25% sulfosalicylic acid is added, to give white precipitate. Sulfosalicylic acid is an alkaloidal reagent and so it neutralizes the positively charged protein to produce precipitation.

### c. Heller's test

To 3 mL of urine, few mL of conc. nitric acid is added to get a white ring at the junction of 2 fluids.

## 3. Ketone Bodies

The excretion of ketone bodies in urine is called ketonuria. This occurs in ketosis where there will be ketonemia and ketonuria. Ketone bodies are acetone, acetoacetic acid and beta hydroxy butyric acid. They are formed in excess when the glucose metabolism is slow (diabetes mellitus) or when there is starvation and fat is used exclusively to give energy.

## Tests for Ketone Bodies

**a. Rothera's test** (for acetone, and acetoacetic acid)
3 mL of urine is saturated with solid ammonium sulfate. Two drops of sodium nitroprusside is added followed by addition of 2 mL of strong ammonia along the sides of the tube to produce a purplish pink ring at the junction of 2 liquids.

**b. Gerhardt's test** (for acetoacetic acid)
To 5 mL of urine, 10 drops of 10% ferric chloride is added to get maximum precipitate of ferric phosphate. Filter and remove the precipitate. To the filtrate, excess of ferric chloride is added to get a purple/port-wine color.

## 4. Blood

a. **Hematuria:** Passing of whole blood including erythrocytes in urine is called hematuria.
Causes for hematuria : Injury to urinary tract or kidney.
: Infection of urinary tract.
: Benign or malignant carcinoma of kidney or urinary tract.
: Enlargement of prostate due to rupture of engorged venous plexus
: Obstruction due to urinary stones.
b. **Hemoglobinuria:** Excretion of free hemoglobin in urine. It is seen in incompatible blood transfusion, malaria, typhoid, hemolytic jaundice.

### Test for Blood in Urine

### Benzidine Test

To a knife point of benzidine, add 1 mL of glacial acetic acid and dissolve it. Then 1 mL of hydrogen peroxide is added and then 1 mL of urine is added and mixed well. Blue or green color develops which turns to brownish black within few minutes. Hb in blood decomposes hydrogen peroxide and liberates oxygen which oxidises benzidine to a colored compound.

## 5. Bile Salts

Bile salts are sodium and potassium salts of glycocholic and taurocholic acids. They are derivatives of cholesterol. Normally they do not enter general circulation and so are absent in normal urine. Bile salts are present in urine of patients having obstructive jaundice.

### Test for Bile Salts

### a. Hay's Test

5 mL of urine and 5 mL of distilled water (Control) are taken in two test tubes each. Little quantity of sulfur powder is sprinkled over the surface of liquid in each tube. Sulfur powder sinks to the bottom of the tube containing urine as the bile salts decrease the surface tension. Sulfur powder floats on the tube containing water (Control).

### b. Pettenkofer's Test

To 5 mL of urine, 5 drops of 5% sucrose solution is added. The tube is kept in an inclined position, and 2–3 mL of concentrated sulfuric acid is poured along the sides of the tube. A red ring is produced. The contents are mixed gently while keeping the tube under running water. The red color spreads throughout the liquid.
This is a less sensitive test than Hay's test.

## 6. Bile Pigments

Bile pigments are bilirubin and biliverdin. They are produced by the breakdown of heme in the reticuloendothelial system. Bilirubin is in unconjugated form soon after it is produced from heme and it gets conjugated with UDP glucuronic acid in liver. Bile contains conjugated bilirubin which is excreted into the intestines. In normal persons bile pigments are not present in urine.

### Test for Bile Pigments

### a. Fouchet's Test

To 3 mL of urine, few crystals of magnesium sulfate are added and dissolved by shaking. 2 mL of 10% barium chloride is added. A white precipitate of barium sulfate is formed. It is filtered by using filter paper. Unfold the filter paper and dry it. Add 1–2 drops of Fouchet's reagent to the precipitate in the filter paper which oxidises the bilirubin to give green colored pigment biliverdin.

### b. Gmelin's Test

5 mL of concentrated nitric acid is taken in a test tube. Urine is taken in a pipette and it is layered over the nitric acid. Green, blue or violet rings are seen at the junction of the liquids.

## 7. Urobilinogen

Urobilinogen is formed from bilirubin in the intestine by bacterial action. No urobilinogen is found in urine in obstructive jaundice. Urobilinogen is increased in hemolytic jaundice and in toxic jaundice.

### Test for Urobilinogen

To 3 mL urine, few crystals of p-dimethylaminobenzaldehyde (Ehrlich Reagent) and 1 mL of hydrochloric acid are added and mixed. A cherry red color is seen if urobilinogen is present in large amount.

## ■ ANALYSIS OF ABNORMAL CONSTITUENTS OF URINE

| Experiment | Observation | Inference |
|---|---|---|
| **1. Benedict's Test for Glucose and Other Reducing Sugars** | | |
| To 5 mL of Benedict's reagent, 8 drops of urine is added and boiled, and cooled. | Green/yellow/red precipitate is obtained. | Shows the presence of reducing sugars in urine. |
| **2. Test for Ketone Bodies Rothera's Test** | | |
| 3 mL of urine is taken in a test tube. This is saturated with ammonium sulfate powder until a little settles at the bottom. 2 drops of freshly prepared 5% solution of sodium nitroprusside is added and mixed. 2 mL of strong ammonia is added slowly along the sides of the tube and the tube is left in a rack for 5 minutes. | Permanganate colored ring is seen at the junction of both liquids. | Shows the presence of ketone bodies in urine. |

*(Contd...)*

*(Contd...)*

| Experiment | Observation | Inference |
|---|---|---|
| **3. Test for Proteins** | | |
| **a. Heat coagulation test** Urine is taken up to 3/4th of a test tube and the upper portion is heated by holding the test tube at the bottom. 3–5 drops of 1% acetic acid is added. | A white precipitate is formed. | Indicates the presence of heat coagulable proteins (Albumin). |
| **b. Sulfosalicylic acid** To 2 mL of urine few drops of 25% sulfosalicylic acid is added. | A white precipitate is formed. | Indicates the presence of proteins in urine. |
| **c. Heller's test** To 3 mL of urine few drops of conc. $HNO_3$ is added | A white ring is formed at the junction of the 2 fluids. | Indicates the presence of proteins in urine. |
| **4. Test for Blood** | | |
| **Benzidine test** A small quantity of Benzidine powder is taken in a knife point and 1 mL of glacial acetic acid is added and mixed. 1 mL of hydrogen peroxide is added to that and mixed. 1 mL of urine is then added. | A blue or green color develops first. Then it changes to black color within few minutes. | Shows the presence of blood in urine. |
| **5. Test for Bile Salt** | | |
| **Hay's test** 2 test tubes are taken. In the first tube 2 mL of urine and in the second tube 2 mL of distilled water are taken. A small quantity of sulfur powder is sprinkled over the surface of the liquid in each tube. | Sulfur powder sinks in the tube containing urine. | Indicates the presence of bile salts. Bile salts reduce the surface tension and hence the sulfur powder sinks to the bottom |
| **6. Test for Bile Pigments** | | |
| **Fouchet's test** To 3 mL of urine few crystals of magnesium sulfate is added and dissolved. Then 2 mL of 10% barium chloride is added and mixed. A white precipitate is formed. It is filtered and the precipitate in the filter paper is dried and 1–2 drops of Fouchet's reagent is added. | A green color develops in the filter paper. | Indicates the presence of bile pigments. The precipitate formed is barium sulfate which absorbs bile pigments. Ferric chloride present in Fouchet's reagent oxidises bilirubin to green colored biliverdin. |

## Relevant Questions

### Normal and Abnormal Urine

1. Name the normal constituents of urine.
2. What is the volume of normal daily urine?
3. What is the normal color of urine due to?
4. What is the normal specific gravity of urine?
5. What is the pH of normal urine?

6. What is the chief anion of urine?
7. What is the normal level of calcium excreted in per day urine?
8. In which diseases calcium will be excreted in large quantities in urine?
9. What is the normal phosphate level in urine? In which disease the level will be increased?
10. What is the level of normal excretion of ammonia?
11. Name the NPN substances present in urine.
12. How much of urea is excreted in per day urine?
13. What is urea?
14. How urea is formed and where is it synthesized?

# CHAPTER 7

# Screening of Urine for Inborn Errors of Metabolism and the Use of Paper Chromatography

**BI11.5** Describe the use of paper chromatography.
**BI11.20** Identify abnormal constituents in urine, interpret the findings and correlate these with pathological states.

## ■ SCREENING OF URINE FOR INBORN ERRORS OF METABOLISM (IEM)

Inborn errors of metabolism are rare genetic or inherited disorders resulting from an enzyme defect in biochemical and metabolic pathways of biomolecules such as carbohydrate, proteins, lipids, etc., causing various disorders in many human organ systems.

The term inborn errors of metabolism was coined by Archibald Garrod who is known as the Father of IEM. Four in born error disorders were found out by him and named as Garrod's tetrad—Essential pentosuria, alkaptonuria, cystinuria and albinism.

Most of the disorders have the following manifestations affecting the major organ systems such as:
- Growth failure, mental retardation
- Developmental delay, seizures
- Deafness, blindness
- Skin pigmentation, dental abnormalities
- Immunodeficiency
- Recurrent vomiting, diarrhea, abdominal pain
- Liver enlargement, jaundice, liver failure
- Unusual facial features, congenital malformations.

## Diagnosis

- These diseases are detectable by—prenatal diagnosis, newborn screening tests, especially using Tandem mass spectrometry (TMS)
- In the laboratory, urinary or blood screening tests can be done to diagnose these disorders and by doing paper chromatography the diagnosis will be confirmed.

Chapter 7: Screening of Urine for Inborn Errors of Metabolism and the Use of Paper Chromatography

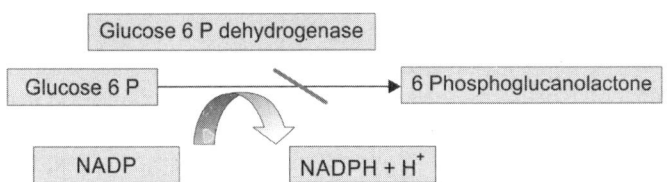

Fig. 7.1: Rate limiting step by G6PD.

# A. CONGENITAL DISORDERS OF CARBOHYDRATE METABOLISM

## 1. Glucose 6 Phosphate Dehydrogenase Deficiency (Fig. 7.1)

- Rate limiting step—catalyzed by glucose-6-phosphate dehydrogenase enzyme which is NADP dependent. One NADPH is produced
- Glucose 6 phosphate dehydrogenase deficiency—Congenital—X-linked recessive trait
- This will lead to drug-induced hemolytic anemia
- The deficiency is manifested only when exposed to certain oxidant drugs or toxins like primaquine for malaria or ingestion of toxic glycosides in Fava beans (favism)
- Sulfa drugs may also precipitate hemolysis. This leads to jaundice and severe anemia
- This disease offers resistance to plasmodium infection and protects the individual from malaria since the parasite requires reduced glutathione which is not available in the G6PD deficiency
- Screening test:
  A. Sodium nitrite and methylene blue reduction test: To a citrated blood sample, sodium nitrite and methylene blue are added. Persistence of brown color indicates deficiency – because in G6PD deficiency, there is deficiency of NADPH and so Hb is oxidized to methemoglobin to give brown color.
  B. Estimation of G6PD in RBC.

## 2. Galactosemia/Galactose Metabolism (Fig.7. 2)

- It is an inborn error of metabolism in galactose metabolism
- Defect: Deficiency of galactose 1 phosphate uridyl transferase enzyme. Inherited defects of galactokinase, uridyl transferase, or 4-epimerase can also cause galactosemia
- Features:
  a. Hypoglycemia: Due to accumulation of galactose 1 P which inhibits galactokinase and glycogen phosphorylase
  b. Enlargement of liver (jaundice)
  c. Severe mental retardation
  d. Congenital cataract: Due to enzyme deficiency, Galactose is reduced to dulcitol which gets accumulated in lens causing cataract due to its osmotic effect
  e. Galactosemia: Due to accumulation of galactose in blood and galactosuria.

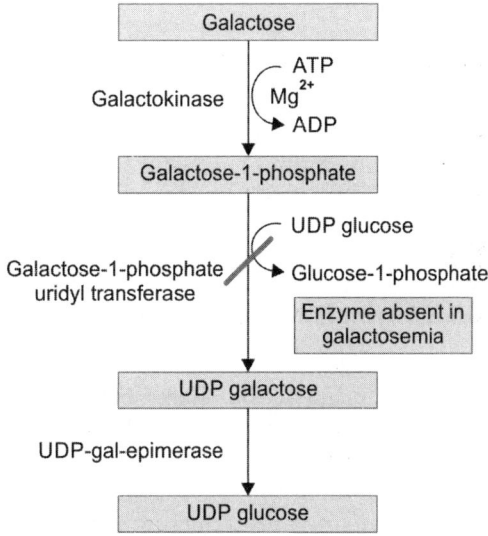

Fig. 7.2: Galactose metabolism.

## Screening Test

- Presence of galactose in urine (galactosuria)—By Benedict's test for reducing sugar—To 5 mL of Benedict's reagent, 8 drops of urine is added and boiled and allowed to cool. Green or yellow or red precipitate is obtained depending upon the amount of reducing sugar present in it.
- To 2 mL of Seliwanoff's reagent, 3 drops of fructose solution is added and boiled for 30 seconds. Then the test tube is allowed to cool in the rack. Cherry red colored complex is not formed which shows the absence of fructose. Fructose is ruled out by this.
- Urine chromatography for galactose.

**Refer Chapter 43—Clinical Case studies—for Q & A**

## 3. Hereditary Fructose Intolerance (Fig.7.3)

- It is an inborn error of fructose metabolism
- Cause: Due to the absence of hepatic **aldolase B,** this cleaves fructose 1-phosphate.

### Hereditary Fructose Intolerance

There will be accumulation of Fructose 1-P which inhibits fructokinase causing impaired clearance of fructose from blood.

### Clinical Features

- Accumulation of F-1-P leads to liver and kidney damage.
- Fructose-induced **hypoglycemia** despite the presence of high glycogen reserve due to inhibition of Glycogenolysis and Gluconeogenesis.

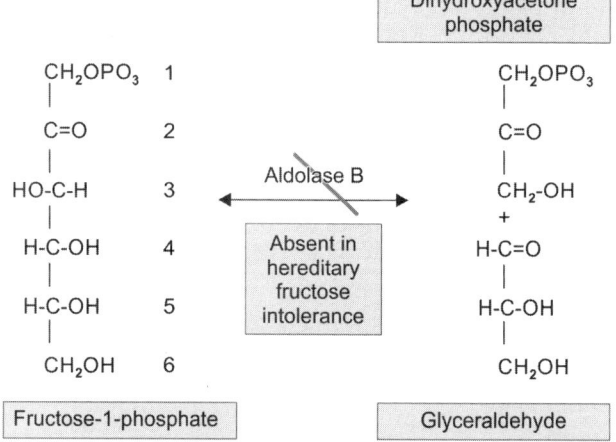

Fig. 7.3: Hereditary fructose intolerance.

## Screening Test

- Positive Benedict's test shows presence of reducing sugar
- Positive Seliwanoff's test—Confirmatory test for fructose
- Chromatography of urine for sugar

**Refer Chapter 43—Clinical Case studies—for Q & A**

## ■ B. CONGENITAL DISORDERS OF PROTEIN METABOLISM

## 4. Phenylketonuria—Classical (Fig. 7.4)

- It is an autosomal recessive disease with an incidence of 1:10,000 births. It is due to deficiency of phenylalanine hydroxylase.
- So phenylalanine is not converted into tyrosine and it accumulates— Hyperphenylalaninemia.

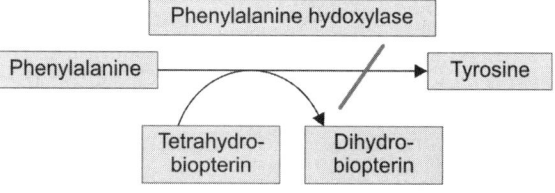

Fig. 7.4: Phenylketonuria: Classical.

## Chapter 7: Screening of Urine for Inborn Errors of Metabolism and the Use of Paper Chromatography

- The excess of phenylalanine is converted to phenyl pyruvate, phenyl lactate, and phenyl acetate and phenylacetylglutamine. Phenyl pyruvate, phenyl lactate, phenyl acetate are excreted in urine.

### *Clinical Manifestations*

- The child is mentally retarded
- Convulsions, tremors, agitation, hyperactivity may be present.
- The child often has hypopigmentation due to reduced availability of tyrosine for melanin production.
- Phenyl lactate in sweat causes mousy body odor.

### *Laboratory Diagnosis*

- Blood level of phenylalanine is elevated—Normal level is 1 mg/dL, which is elevated to >20 mg/dL.
- This is confirmed by Tandem mass spectroscopy
- Guthrie's test is confirmative: In blood
- Urine:
  a. *Ferric chloride test*: To one mL of urine 2 drops of ferric chloride solution is added. Few drops of sulfuric acid are then added dropwise. Dark green colour indicates positive test.
  b. *DNPH test (Dinitrophenylhydrazine test)*: 2 mL of urine is added to 2 mL of DNPH reagent and mixed well and after 10 minutes yellow precipitate is formed-which shows the test is positive.
- DNA probes—to diagnose the defects in phenylalanine hydroxylase and dihydrobiopterin reductase
- Paper chromatography—for amino acids

**Refer Chapter 43—Clinical Case studies—for Q & A**

## 5. Alkaptonuria (Fig. 7.5)

- It is an inborn error of metabolism of Tyrosine/Phenylalanine—it is a harmless condition
- It is an autosomal recessive condition – of Garrod's tetrad
- It is due to the defect in homogentisate oxidase enzyme
- Homogentisate gets accumulated and oxidised to benzoquinone acetate and forms alkaptone bodies
- Alkaptone bodies get deposited in intervertebral discs, cartilages of nose and pinna of ear developing Ochronosis. Black pigments get deposited over joint cavities causing arthritis.

### *Screening Test*

**Urine:**

- Urine turns black on standing
- $FeCl_3$ test is positive. Refer Phenylketonuria

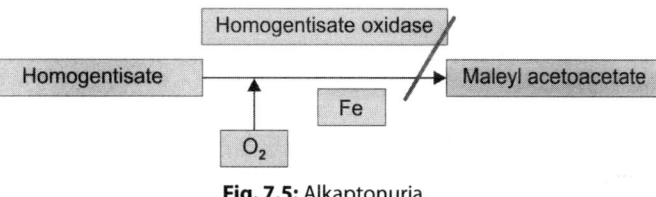

**Fig. 7.5:** Alkaptonuria.

- Benedict's test is strongly positive since homogentisate is a reducing agent
- Paper chromatography—for amino acids

**Refer Chapter 43—Clinical Case studies—for Q & A**

## 6. Maple Syrup Urinary Disease (MSUD) (Fig. 7.6)

- This is also known as branched chain ketonuria
- This is due to the deficiency of the enzyme branched chain keto acid dehydrogenase—the second enzyme in the catabolism of branched chain amino acids such as valine, leucine and isoleucine.

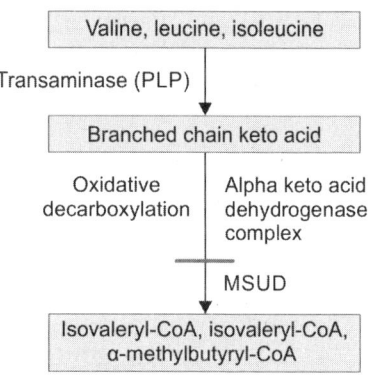

**Fig. 7.6:** Maple syrup urinary disease.

### Clinical Features

- Symptoms start from the first week of birth.
- It is characterized by mental retardation, convulsions, vomiting, acidosis, coma and death within first year of life.
- The urine smells like burnt sugar or maple syrup. Urine contains branched chain keto acids, valine, Leucine or isoleucine.
- Rothera's test—positive.

## 7. Homocystinurias (Fig. 7.7)

- These are the inborn errors of metabolism in methionine metabolism. These are autosomal recessive disorders.
- Normal homocysteine level in blood is 5–15 micromol/L. It is highly increased in disease conditions. In elderly people in vitamin $B_6$ or $B_{12}$ deficiency, smokers, alcoholics and in hypothyroidism also the level is increased. Large amounts of homocystine are excreted in urine in these conditions
- Hyperhomocysteinemia is a risk factor for coronary heart disease. It is seen in smokers, alcoholics, and hypothyroidism.

Congenital Homocystinurias are due to:
1. Cystathionine beta synthase deficiency: Type I
2. Deficient $N^5$, $N^{10}$ Methylene THFA reductase: Type II
3. Cobalamin deficiency: Type III
4. Defective intestinal absorption of Vitamin $B_{12}$: Type IV

### 1. Cystathionine Beta Synthase Deficiency

- Methionine and homocysteine levels are increased in blood and in urine.
- Marked decrease in plasma cysteine level.

### Clinical Features

- Mental retardation, Charlie Chaplin gait, skeletal deformities and Ectopia lentis in eyes are seen

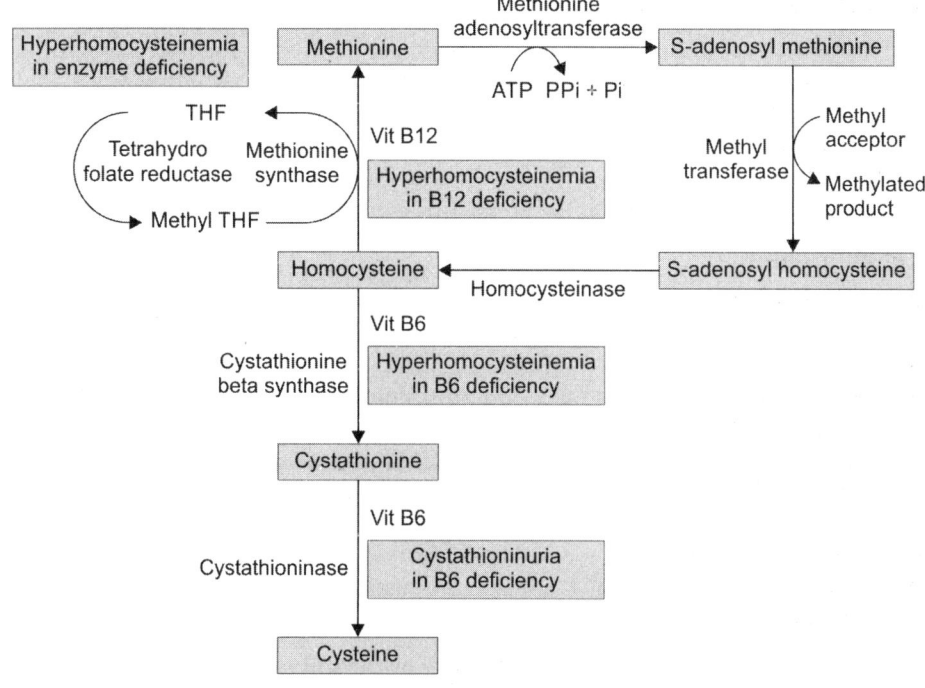

**Fig. 7.7:** Methionine metabolism.

- Homocysteine activates Hageman's factor causing platelet aggregation leading to intravascular thrombosis.

## Urine

- **Cyanide nitroprusside test:** 5 drops of urine is taken in a watch glass and a drop of ammonium hydroxide and 2 drops of sodium cyanide are added and mixed. 1 drop of 1% sodium nitroprusside is added after 10 minutes—Deep red color shows positive test for cystine and homocystine.
- Urinary homocysteine are elevated.
- Normal homocysteine level in blood is 5–15 mmol/L. It is increased up to 50–100 times in homocystinuria.

### 2. Cobalamin Deficiency

$N^5$ methyl THFA homocysteine methyl transferase is dependent on $B_{12}$. So in $B_{12}$ deficiency, Homocysteine cannot be converted to methionine. Hence hyperhomocysteinemia occurs.

### 3. Deficient $N^5$, $N^{10}$ Methylene THFA Reductase

- This leads to reduced methionine synthesis with increase in homocysteine level in urine
- There will be behavioral changes and vascular abnormalities.

## Chromatographic separations

i. Separation of aminoacids in urine by paper chromatography (Refer Ch. 25).
ii. Separation of sugars in urine by paper chromatography

## Technique of Separation of Sugar in Urine

- First Pyridine extract of the urine to be analyzed is prepared as follows: 10 mL of urine is heated over water bath to dryness. 2 mL of pyridine is added to it and stirred well. It is left to stand for sometime and then centrifuged and used.
- Take a Whatman No.1 filter paper of dimensions appropriate (14" × 12") for the chromatographic chamber (bell jar) used. Draw a line with a pencil along the width of the paper 5 cm from its edge. Mark points on the line 2 cm from the edge at distances of 2 cm.

## Application of sample:

- **Test:** 20 mL of pyridine extract of urine (equivalent to 100 mL of urine) is applied with the graduated micropipette—1 cm apart- 0.5 cm in diameter and 1.5 cm from the bottom of the sheet.
- **Standard:** 20 mL each of 2 separate standard solutions—one with glucose and lactose in 100 mL of water and another containing 100 mg of galactose in 100 mL of water are run along with the test for reference and developed in the solvent—Butanol/Ethyl alcohol/Pyridine/Aq—in the proportion of 30/30/25/20 v/v and place it in a shallow trough and cover it with the bell jar.
- After the development the paper is dried for 30 minutes and sprayed with Benzidine reagent and heated for five minutes at 110°C. Presence of sugar is indicated by brown spots on a light yellow background.

$$Rf = \frac{\text{Distance travelled by the solute}}{\text{Distance travelled by the solvent}}$$

- Distance travelled by solute = Distance from the center of the spot applied to the center of the spot migrated.
- Distance travelled by solvent = Distance from the pencil line to the marked solvent front.

# CHAPTER 8

# Composition of Cerebrospinal Fluid

**BI11.15** Describe and discuss the composition of CSF.

## ■ CEREBROSPINAL FLUID (CSF)

It is found in the subarachnoid space, ventricles of brain and in the spinal cord. It originates in the choroid plexus. The total volume of CSF is 125 mL. It is a transudate.

## Collection of CSF (Fig. 8.1)

Cerebrospinal fluid is collected by a procedure called lumbar puncture. A sterile lumbar puncture needle is introduced between the L3 and L4 vertebra under strict aseptic precautions with the patient lying in lateral position. After the puncture, the cerebrospinal fluid is gently allowed to flow and collected in sterile bottles for analysis.

## Normal Composition of CSF

1. Color and appearance: Clear colorless
2. Cell count: $0.4 \times 10^6/L$
3. Protein: 15–40 mg/dL
4. Sugar: 50–70 mg/dL
   - CSF Glucose decreased in bacterial meningitis, tuberculous meningitis.
   - CSF Proteins: (albumin: 20 mg/dL, Globulin 5–10 mg/dL).

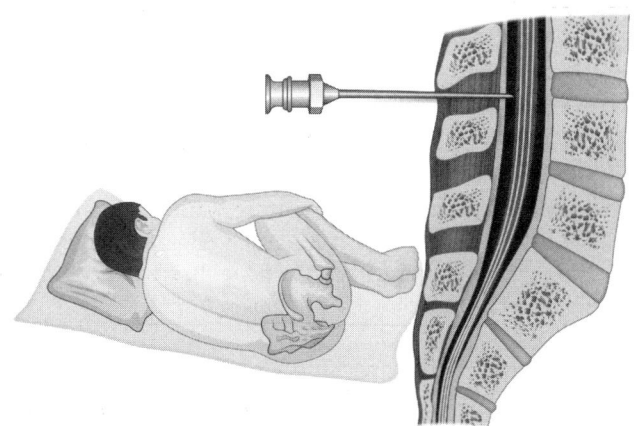

**Fig. 8.1:** Lumbar puncture for CSF collection.

## CSF Increased in:

- Bacterial—meningitis (marked increase). tuberculous meningitis
- Viral fever, brain tumor
- Subarachnoid hemorrhage.

## Analysis of Cerebrospinal Fluid

The chemical analysis of CSF consists in the estimation for protein, sugar and chloride. The protein content of CSF is usually low and hence is determined by measuring the turbidity produced when sulfosalicylic acid is added. Sugar is estimated by GOD-POD method. Chloride is estimated by Ion selective electrode method.

### 1. Analysis of Proteins

**Procedure:** Mark three test tubes S, T and B for standard, test and blank respectively. Proceed as follows:

| Reagents | Standard (mL) | Test (mL) | Blank (mL) |
|---|---|---|---|
| Standard Protein | 1.0 | — | — |
| CSF | — | 1.0 | — |
| 0.9 % NaCl | — | — | 1.0 |
| 3% sulfosalicylic acid | 4.0 | 4.0 | 4.0 |

Mix the contents of each tube and wait for 5 minutes. Set water at zero at 450 nm (blue filter) Read the OD of Blank, Standard and Test.

Concentration of standard protein: 50 mg%.

### Calculation

- Amount of protein in the given CSF sample = $\dfrac{ODT-ODB}{ODS-ODB} \times \dfrac{1.5}{1.0} \times 100 \, mg$

- Analysis of 24 hours urine protein—Similar to CSF protein.
- Analysis of other body fluids protein (ascitic, peritoneal, pleural, etc.). Similar to that of total plasma proteins by Biuret method.

### 2. Analysis of Chloride

It is possible to titrate CSF chloride directly with silver nitrate solution using potassium dichromate as indicator:
- The reagents used are silver nitrate solution and potassium chromate 10% solution.
- 1 mL of CSF is added with 2.5 mL of distilled water and add 1 drop of potassium chromate.
- Titrate with silver nitrate to the usual brick red color. Repeat the titrations for confirmation.
- Calculate the chloride level in 100 mL of CSF.

### 3. Estimation of Glucose

Glucose level in CSF is estimated as per the method used in blood sugar estimation.

### 4. Test for Globulins

**Pandy's test**: Add 2 drops of CSF to 2 mL of reagent (10 g phenol + 150 mL water). Note the degree of opalescence or turbidity. Marked opalescence or turbidity is indicative of increased globulins seen in multiple sclerosis and neurosyphilis.

# SECTION 3

# Quantitative Experiments

## Section Outline

9. Principles of Colorimetry
10. Principles of Spectrophotometer
11. Estimation of Glucose
12. Glucose Tolerance Test
13. Estimation of Serum and Urine Creatinine: Creatinine Clearance
14. Estimation of Urea
15. Serum Proteins—Albumin: Globulin Ratio
16. Serum Total Cholesterol
17. Lipid Profile
18. Serum Calcium and Phosphorus
19. Serum Bilirubin
20. Serum Transaminases
21. Serum Alkaline Phosphatase
22. Serum of Uric Acid

# CHAPTER 9

# Principles of Colorimetry

**BI11.6** Describe the principles of colorimetry.

## ■ COLORIMETRY (ABSORPTION PHOTOMETRY)

Most widely used technique in biochemical estimations. Colorimetry is the measurement of colors. So the substance to be estimated colorimetrically should be either colored or capable of forming chromogens by the addition of reagents. The instrument used is called colorimeter. It acts as an absorptiometer by measuring the amount of light absorbed by the colored substance.

## Principle

Colored solutions have the property of absorbing certain wave lengths of light and transmitting others. This property is based on Beer-Lambert's law.

## Beer's Law

When monochromatic light passes through a colored solution, the amount of light transmitted decreases exponentially with the increase in concentration of the colored substance. In other words, the intensity of the color is directly proportionate to the concentration of the colored particle in solution.

## Lambert's Law

The amount of light transmitted decreases exponentially with increase in the thickness of the layer of the colored solution. The amount of light absorbed by the colored solution depends on the length of the column or depth of the liquid through which light passes.

Combining these two principles, Beer-Lambert's law can be expressed as:

$$\frac{I_e}{I_0} = e^{-kct}$$

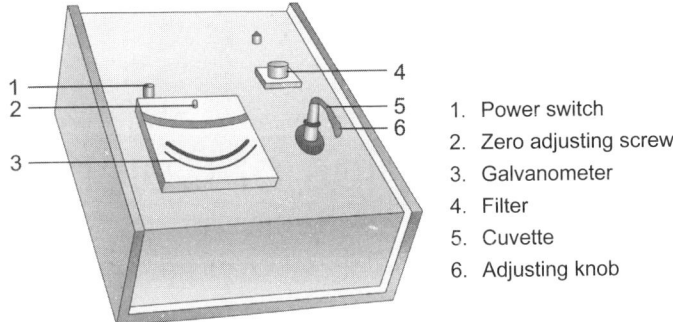

**Fig. 9.1:** Photoelectric colorimeter.

## Photoelectric Colorimeter (Fig. 9.1)

$I_e$ = Intensity of emergent light
k = Constant
$I_0$ = Intensity of incident light
c = Concentration of colored substance
t = Thickness or length of the layer or column through which light passes
The ratio is called transmittance (T).

Percentage $\frac{I_e}{I_0}$ of transmission is given by $\frac{I_e}{I_0} \times 100$. The absorbance is expressed as $-\log T$.

## Optical Density (OD)

It is $-\log T$. Optical density (OD) is the term used in colorimetry for expressing the reading. As it is a logarithmic scale, values too low or too high are not acceptable for accurate results. (sensitive range is 0.1–0.6)

## Parts of Colorimeter (Fig. 9.2)

1. Source of light—filament lamp
2. Monochromatic filters

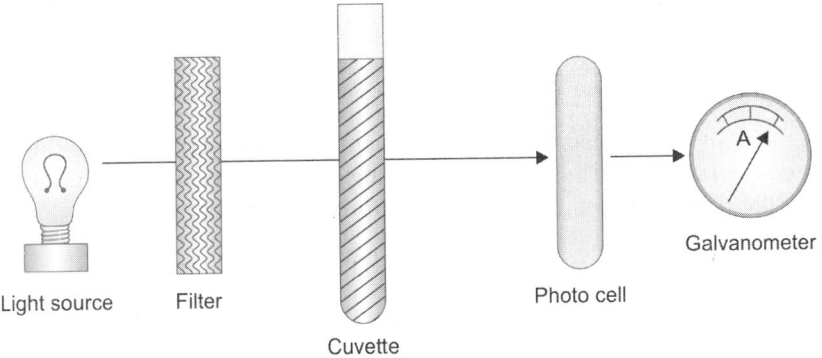

**Fig. 9.2:** Parts of colorimeter.

3. Cuvette—sample holder (small glass tubes)
4. Photo cell—Detector
5. Display—Galvanometer (or digital).

## Filters

Filters will absorb light of unwanted wavelength and allow only monochromatic light to pass through. This light will have maximum absorbance when passed through a particular colored solution.

The monochromatic light after passing the filter is allowed to fall on the colored solution kept in the cuvette. The solution absorbs part of the light and the remaining light is allowed to fall on the photo cells which convert light into an electrical signal. The electrical signal generated is directly proportional to the intensity of the light falling on the detector. These signals are measured by a galvanometer and read as absorbance or optical density (OD) values.

| Color of filters (Color absorbed) | Wavelength of absorption (Nanometer) | Color of solution (Complementary color) |
|---|---|---|
| • Violet | • 420 (400–435) | • Brown |
| • Blue | • 470 (435–495) | • Yellow-Brown |
| • Blue Green | • 490 (490–500) | • Orange Red |
| • Green | • 520 (500–560) | • Pink |
| • Yellow | • 580 (560–580) | • Purple (Violet) |
| • Orange | • 600 (590–650) | • Blue Green |
| • Red | • 680 (650–700) | • Green |

## Procedure

In all colorimetric analysis it is necessary to prepare 3 solutions namely a blank (distilled water), test (specified volume of the blood filtrate or other specimens) and a standard. The standard solution is prepared by treating a solution of the pure substance of known concentration. A standard graph with different concentrations should be prepared.

The appropriate colored filter is chosen and the cuvette is filled to about three fourth with distilled water and placed in the cuvette slot. Instrument is switched on and allowed to warm up for 4–5 minutes. Zero optic density should be adjusted first. Now the distilled water should be removed and the solution in the test tube labelled 'blank' should be taken in the cuvette and OD is read and noted. Similarly, OD for test and standard solution are read and noted.

## Calculation

$$\text{Concentration of the test solution} = \frac{\text{OD of Test (T)}}{\text{OD of Std (S)}} - \frac{\text{OD of Blank (B)}}{\text{OD of Blank (B)}} \times \frac{\text{Conc. of Std}}{\text{Vol. of Test}} \times 100$$

$$= \frac{T-B}{S-B} \times \frac{\text{Conc. of Std}}{\text{Vol. of Test}}$$

## End-point Analysis

Serum sample and reagents are mixed, incubated at 37°C for a fixed time (10–15 min) to develop color optimally. After the incubation period, OD is ascertained and concentration of substance is calculated.

## Kinetic Analysis

Serum and reagents are incubated, and readings taken at 2 and 3 min exactly. The concentration is calculated by the difference in OD between the 2 values. Here no optimal color is developed but it is a quicker method. So, it is used in autoanalyzers.

# CHAPTER 10

# Principles of Spectrophotometer

**BI11.18** Discuss the principles of Spectrophotometry.

## ■ SPECTROPHOTOMETER

Spectrophotometry is a technique which measures absorption and transmission of light over a certain range of wavelength. The instrument which is based on this is called spectrophotometer. It works on the same principle of colorimeter (**Fig. 10.1**).

## Parts

1. **Source of light:** Tungsten lamp—to get visible spectrum and deuterium lamp to get UV spectrum.
2. **Monochromators:** Either prisms or gratings
3. **Cuvettes:** Quartz or fused silica.
4. **Detectors:** To measure light intensity by converting light signal to electric signal. The detectors commonly used are barrier layer cells and photo multiplier tubes.
5. **Galvanometer:** Reading device.

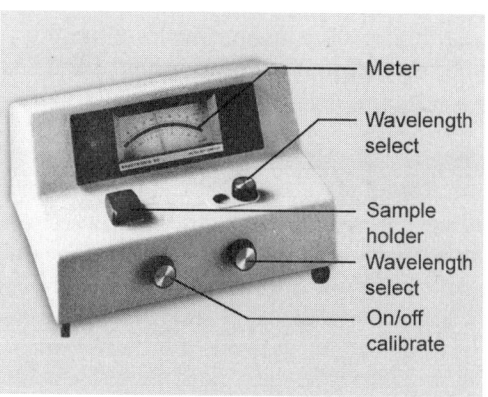

**Fig. 10.1:** Spectrophotometer.

## Types

1. Single beam spectrophotometer.
2. Double beam spectrophotometer.

## Single Beam Spectrophotometer

It records the ratio of the incident beam energy to the transmitted beam energy. The absorbance is the logarithm of the ratio which is obtained by taking the reading at the detector with no sample in the light path. A beam splitter or a pulsed light source is used for the ratio recording.

### *Advantages of Single Beam*
- Improved transmission of light—result by less number of optical components
- Greater sensitivity due to higher light throughput.

## Double Beam Spectrophotometer

Here the incident beam is split into two portions. One portion passes through the sample and the other through the blank reference. The ratio of the two beams is recorded by the detector in real time.

### *Advantages of Double Beam*
- Fluctuations in lamp energy occurs in single beam between the recording measurements can be prevented
- Correction of absorbance in solvent blank
- Correction due to fluctuation in beam intensity variations, stray light and electronic noise are applied in real time.

## Applications and Uses of Spectrophotometer
- Routine analysis in clinical chemistry of enzymes and other routine parameters
- Identification of compounds in pure state and in biological mixtures
- Determination of conformational changes in protein
- Monitoring reactions involved in catalytic chromophores
- Measurement of compounds at the characteristic absorption wavelength, e,g., Proteins –220 nm; Tryptophan –280 nm.

# CHAPTER 11

# Estimation of Glucose

**BI11.17** Explain the basis and rationale of biochemical tests done in the following conditions:
- Diabetes mellitus
- Dyslipidemia
- Myocardial infarction
- Renal failure, Gout
- Proteinuria
- Nephrotic syndrome
- Edema
- Jaundice
- Liver diseases, pancreatitis
- Acid base disorders
- Thyroid disorders

**BI11.21** Demonstrate estimation of glucose, creatinine, urea and total protein in serum.

## ■ DEMONSTRATION AND ESTIMATION

### 1. Estimation of Blood Glucose

The term blood sugar denotes mainly glucose—the sugar of the body. There are many methods to estimate the level of glucose in blood.

**I. Manual methods (colorimetric)**
1. Enzymatic methods
   - Glucose oxidase peroxidase (GOD/POD) method.
   - This gives the true value of glucose.
2. Methods depending on the reducing property of glucose
   (Value is 5–20 mg% higher due to the presence of non-glucose reducing substances like glutathione, ergothioneine in RBCs, glucuronic acid and its compounds, urates and ascorbate).
   a. Alkaline copper reduction methods
      - Folin-Wu method: Proteins precipitated by tungstic acid. Reduced copper is estimated by reacting with phosphomolybdic acid.
      - Modified Folin-Wu method (method of Asatoor and King): More stable color is produced.

b. **Ferricyanide reduction methods**
Reduction of ferricyanide to ferrocyanide in alkaline media and the amount of ferrocyanide is measured.
3. **O-Toluidine method**
The color given by aldoses with O-Toluidine in glacial acetic acid is measured. Expensive method. O-Toluidine should be used carefully as it is a carcinogenic substance.
II. **Autoanalyzer methods:** Mainly by glucose oxidase peroxidase methods (GOD/POD).
III. **Titration method using Iodimetry**
IV. **Solid phase tests for glucose (dry chemistry)**
 - Using Dextrostix and color compared
 - Visidex II in strips.
V. **Glucometer**
 - Choice of blood specimen:
    1. Capillary blood from thumb or a finger: Capillary blood glucose is 20–35 mg% higher than the venous blood.
    2. Venous blood: Postprandial blood sugar is 20–30 mg% higher in arterial blood than in venous blood.
    3. Plasma or serum glucose level is slightly higher than the whole blood.
 - **Preservative used** (anticoagulant—antiglycolytic preservatives)
   Sodium fluoride and potassium oxalate mixture (20 mg/5 mL) in the ratio of 1:3 is suitable.
   NaF—Inhibits conversion of 2-phosphoglycerate to phosphoenolpyruvate by inhibiting enolase enzyme thereby preventing glycolysis.
   Potassium oxalate—acts as an anticoagulant.

## A-1. Modified Folin-Wu Method

**Principle:** Proteins of blood are precipitated with tungstic acid. The clear protein free filtrate containing glucose is heated with alkaline copper solution. Cupric sulfate present in the alkaline copper solution is reduced to cuprous oxide by glucose which is a reducing sugar. On addition of phosphomolybdic acid, the cuprous oxide is oxidised to cupric and the molybdic acid is reduced to molybdenum blue and its color is measured colorimetrically using red filter at 620 nm. The intensity of the blue color is proportionate to the amount of glucose present.

### Folin-Wu Tube (Fig. 11.1)

This tube has got a long stem with 2 graduated marks with a constricted neck which ends in a bulb.

### Advantages

- It provides more stable solution.
- It minimizes reoxidation of cuprous oxide by atmospheric oxygen before adding phosphomolybdic acid.

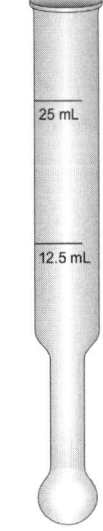

**Fig. 11.1:** Folin-Wu tube.

## Reagents Required

1. 10% Sodium tungstate
2. 2/3 N Conc. Sulfuric acid
3. Alkaline copper reagent—Containing:
   - Anhydrous sodium carbonate
   - Tartaric acid—Copper Sulfate
4. Phosphomolybdic acid—Containing:
   - Sodium tungstate, Molybdic acid
   - 10% sodium hydroxide, Orthophosphoric acid.
5. Standard glucose solution:
   a. Stock standard: 1 g% in saturated Benzoic acid
   b. Working standard: 10 mL of Stock solution in 100 mL of distilled water.
6. Distilled water.

## Procedure

### Preparation of Protein-free Filtrate

Take 3 centrifuge tubes and label them as B (Blank), T (Test) and S (Standard) and proceed as shown in the tabular column.

| Reagent | Blank (mL) | Std (mL) | Test (mL) |
| --- | --- | --- | --- |
| Distilled water | 3.6 | 3.4 | 3.4 |
| Blood sample | — | — | 0.2 |
| Working Glucose standard | — | 0.2 | — |
| 10% Sodium tungstate | 0.2 | 0.2 | 0.2 |
| 2/3N Sulfuric acid | 0.2 | 0.2 | 0.2 |
| **Total** | 4 | 4 | 4 |

Mix well. Allow to stand for 5 minutes. Centrifuge the tubes to get a clear filtrate.

Take 3 Folin-Wu sugar tubes. Label them as B (Blank), S (Standard), and T (Test) and proceed as follows:

| Reagent | Blank (mL) | Standard (mL) | Test (mL) |
| --- | --- | --- | --- |
| Filtrate | 1.0 | 1.0 | 1.0 |
| Alkaline Copper Reagent | 1.0 | 1.0 | 1.0 |
| Mix well. Keep the tubes in boiling water bath for exactly 8 minutes. Cool to room temperature and then add. | | | |
| Phosphomolybdic acid | 1.0 | 1.0 | 1.0 |

Distilled water: upto 12.5 mL mark in each tube

Invert the tubes by placing the mouth of the tube tightly over the palm and mix the contents thoroughly. Repeat it for all the 3 tubes. Read the optical density of the all 3 solutions in a photoelectric colorimeter using 620 nm (red filter).

**Calculation:** Using the general formula for colorimetry.

$$\text{Conc. of glucose in mg/100 mL} = \frac{\text{Test OD} - \text{Blank OD}}{\text{Std OD} - \text{Blank OD}} \times \frac{\text{Conc. of Std}}{\text{Vol. of Sample in filtrate}} \times 100$$

$$= \frac{\text{OD T} - \text{B}}{\text{OD S} - \text{B}} \times 100 \text{ mg}$$

## A-2. Estimation of Blood Glucose by Folin-Wu Method (Using Readymade Protein Free Filtrate)

### Principle

Proteins of blood are precipitated with fresh tungstic acid. The clear protein free filtrate containing glucose is heated with alkaline copper sulfate solution. Cupric sulfate present in the alkaline copper solution is reduced to cuprous oxide by glucose which is a reducing sugar. On addition of phosphomolybdic acid, the cuprous oxide is oxidised to cupric and the molybdic acid is reduced to molybdenum blue and its color is measured colorimetrically using red filter at 620 nm. The intensity of the color is proportional to the amount of glucose present.

### Reagents Required

1. Protein free filtrate.
2. Alkaline copper solution containing anhydrous sodium carbonate and tartaric acid and copper sulfate.
3. Phosphomolybdic acid containing sodium tungstate, molybdic acid and 10% sodium hydroxide and orthophosphoric acid.
4. Stock standard—1 g in 100 mL of saturated benzoic acid.
   Working standard 10 mL of stock standard diluted to 100 mL with distilled water—100 mg%.

### Procedure

Take 3 long Folin-Wu tubes. Mark them as Blank (B), Standard (S) and Test (T)

| Reagents | Blank (mL) | Standard (mL) | Test (mL) |
|---|---|---|---|
| Distilled water | 1.0 | — | — |
| Protein free filtrate | — | — | 1.0 |
| Working standard | — | 1.0 | — |
| Alkaline copper reagent | 1.0 | 1.0 | 1.0 |
| Mix well. Keep them in boiling water bath for exactly 8 minutes. Cool to room temperature and then add 1 mL of phosphomolybdic acid | | | |
| Phosphomolybdic acid | 1.0 | 1.0 | 1.0 |

Make up the volume to 12.5 mL in each tube with distilled water. Take the reading at 620 nm red filter in a photoelectric colorimeter.

## Calculation

Concentration of glucose in 100 mL of filtrate =

$$\frac{OD(T) - OD(B)}{OD(S) - OD(B)} \times \frac{\text{Concentration of standard}}{\text{Actual volume of blood}} \times 100$$

$$= \frac{T-B}{S-B} \times \frac{0.05}{0.05} \times 100 \text{ mg\%}$$

## Conc. of Standard

- Stock standard Conc.: 1000 mg%
- Working standard: 100 mg%
- 100 mL contains: 100 mg%
- Per 0.2 mL of standard contains: 0.2 mg%
- Total amount of filtrate: 4.0 mL
- 4.0 mL of filtrate contains: 0.2 mg
- Per 1 mL of filtrate contains: $0.2 \times 1/4 = 0.05$ mg

## Actual Volume of Blood

- Actual volume of blood taken: 0.2 mL
- 4.0 mL of filtrate is from: 0.2 mL blood
- Per 1 mL of filtrate contains: $0.2 \times 1/4 = 0.05$ mL blood

$$\frac{\text{Conc. of Standard}}{\text{Actual volume of Blood}} \times 100 = \frac{0.05}{0.05} \times 100 = 100$$

# B. Glucose Oxidase Peroxidase (GOD/POD) Method (Manual and Autoanalyzer Method)

## Principle

Glucose is oxidized by glucose oxidase (GOD) to give gluconic acid and hydrogen peroxide. The hydrogen peroxide formed is broken down by peroxidase to water and oxygen. The later oxidizes phenol which combines with 4-aminophenazone to give a red colored complex. The intensity of the red colored complex is proportional to the concentration of glucose in the test. The intensity of the colored complex is measured colorimetrically at 515 nm (500–530).

## Reagents

1. Glycozyme reagent I (Enzyme—chromogen tablets)
2. Glucozyme reagent II (Phenol solution)
3. Glucozyme standard 100 mg/dL.

Glucozyme working reagent is prepared by dissolving one tablet of reagent 1 in 49 mL distilled water to which 1 mL of reagent II (Phenol solution) is added to make final volume 50 mL.

| Reagents | Blank (B) | Standard (S) | Test (T) |
|---|---|---|---|
| Glucozyme working reagent | 1.0 mL | 1.0 mL | 1.0 mL |
| Serum or plasma | — | — | 0.01 mL |
| Standard | — | 0.01 mL | — |
| Distilled water | 0.01 mL | — | — |

Mix the contents of the test tubes thoroughly, and place them in a water bath at 37°C for 15 minutes or at 25°C + 5°C for 30 minutes.

Measure the optical density (OD) of the test and the standard against blank at 515 nm (range 500–530). The final color complex is stable for more than two hours at room temperature.

## Calculation

Glucose present in 100 mL of plasma or serum

$$= \frac{OD(T)-OD(B)}{OD(S)-OD(B)} = \frac{OD(T-B)}{OD(S-B)} \times \text{Concentration of Standard}$$

$$= \frac{OD(T-B)}{OD(T-B)} \times 100 = (\text{Glucose concentration mg/dL})$$

$$= \ldots\ldots\ldots \text{ mg}$$

**Report:** Glucose present in 100 mL of Serum/plasma = ……………………… mg.

## Normal Level of Glucose

- Fasting: 70–110 mg%
- Random: 80–120 mg%
- Postprandial: 90–140 mg%

### HbA1c
It is glycated hemoglobin, which is a nonenzymatic addition of glucose to hemoglobin. Normally the level is less than 6%. It reveals the mean glucose level over the previous 10–12 weeks.

## Clinical Interpretations

1. Hyperglycemia (Increased blood sugar): Found in—
   a. Diabetes mellitus
   b. Cushing's syndrome (Adrenocortical hyperactivity)
   c. Hyperthyroidism
   d. Hyperpituitarism—Acromegaly, gigantism.
   e. Emotional Stress (small increase)
   f. Infections
   g. Intracranial diseases—meningitis, tumors etc.
   h. Effect of drugs—corticosteroids, estrogens, alcohol, etc.

2. Hypoglycemia (Decreased blood sugar values): Found in—
   a. Starvation
   b. Hyperinsulinism
      i. Increased dose of insulin while treating diabetes mellitus.
      ii. Insulin secreting tumors of pancreas
   c. Hypothyroidism (myxedema, cretinism)
   d. Hypopituitarism (e.g. Simmond's disease)
   e. Hypoadrenalism (Addison's disease)
   f. Severe exertion
   g. In children—glycogen storage diseases.
      (e.g.) von Gierke's disease (congenital inherited diseases).

## Relevant Questions

1. What is the normal value of blood glucose level?
2. Name the conditions in which the level is increased?
3. Name the conditions in which blood glucose level is decreased?
4. What are the methods by which blood glucose level can be measured in the laboratory?
5. By which method have you estimated the test?
6. What is the principle of this procedure?
7. Why should you use the specific Folin-Wu sugar tube?
8. What is the color you produced due to?
9. At what wavelength you took the reading?
10. What is the color of the filter you used?
11. What are the components of alkaline copper reagent?

# CHAPTER 12

# Glucose Tolerance Test

> **BI11.19** Outline the basic principles involved in the functioning of instruments commonly used in biochemistry laboratory and their applications.

**Glucose tolerance test (GTT)** is a well standardized test which is highly useful to diagnose diabetes mellitus in doubtful cases. The ability of a person to metabolize a given load of glucose is referred to as glucose tolerance. Usually an oral glucose tolerance test is performed in the clinical laboratory.

## Indications

1. Patient has suggestive symptoms of diabetes mellitus but has inconclusive values of fasting blood sugar.
2. During pregnancy—excessive weight gaining, past history of big baby or miscarriage.
3. To rule out benign renal glycosuria.

**Preparation of patient:** The patient is instructed:
1. To take normal carbohydrate diet for three days prior to the test.
2. To avoid drugs which influence the blood glucose level at least for two days prior to the test.
3. Not to do strenuous exercise on the previous day.
4. Not to take food after 8 PM the previous night to ensure 12 hours fasting.
5. Not to smoke during the test.
6. To report at the laboratory at 8 AM sharp in empty stomach.

## Procedure

A sample of blood (2 mL) and urine sample are collected in the fasting state. Then the patient is given a glucose load of 75 grams dissolved in a glass of water, which he should drink slowly. The glucose water may be flavored to reduce the tendency to vomit. The blood and urine samples are collected at half an hour intervals for the next two and a half hours. Glucose is estimated in all blood samples and urine samples are tested for glucose by Benedict's qualitative test. A graph is plotted with blood glucose concentration on the Y-axis and the time in hours in the X-axis.

## Normal GTT (Fig. 12.1)
1. Fasting blood sugar value is between 80 mg% and 100 mg%.
2. The glucose level rises sharply and a peak is reached at one hour.
3. The blood glucose level comes to normal in two hours.
4. All the urine samples are negative for glucose.

## Renal Glycosuria (Fig. 12.2)
1. It resembles the normal curve.
2. Blood glucose level is not high but glucose is present in all the urine samples. This is due to the lowering of the renal threshold which is seen physiologically in pregnancy, and pathologically in renal tubular defects.

## Impaired Glucose Tolerance (IGT) (Fig.12.3)
1. It is a condition when blood glucose values are above the normal level but below the diabetic level.
2. Fasting blood glucose level is less than 120 mg%.
3. Peak level is above the renal threshold, i.e. higher than 180 mg% at one hour.
4. The blood glucose level comes down in 2 hours to less than 180 mg%.
5. Urine glucose is positive at one hour.
6. IGT patients have associated problems like hypertension, lipid disorders, high uric acid level and obesity.

## Diabetes Mellitus (Fig.12.4)
1. Fasting blood sugar is less than 180 mg% (below the renal threshold value—180 mg%).
2. Peak value is above the renal threshold value.
3. Blood glucose level does not come to the fasting level in two hours and it is more than 180 mg%.
4. All the urine samples are positive for glucose except for the first sample (fasting).

## Gestational Diabetes Mellitus
Gestational diabetes mellitus (GDM) is defined by abnormal glucose tolerance during pregnancy. The glucose tolerance test is normal before and after pregnancy.

## High-risk Patients
1. GDM in previous pregnancy.
2. Family history of diabetes.
3. Previous pregnancy—large weight baby, stillborn infants with congenital abnormalities.
4. Bad obstetric history—hypertension, eclampsia, hydramnios.
5. Obesity.

## Diagnosis of GDM*

100 g of glucose is given and 3 hr GTT** is done.

| Time (hour) | Blood glucose mg/100 mL |
|---|---|
| Fasting 0 | 90 |
| 1 hour | 165 |
| 2 hours | 145 |
| 3 hours | 125 |

Two or more of the above values must be net or exceeded—Diagnostic of gestational diabetes.

*GDM is different from women with diabetes mellitus who become pregnant.
**GTT should not be done if a patient has fasting blood glucose level >140 mg% or 2 hours postprandial level >200 mg%.

## Types of GTT

1. Oral
2. Intravenous (for suspected cases of malabsorption)
3. Corticosteroid stressed GTT to detect any latent diabetes.

## ■ GLUCOSE TOLERANCE TEST CURVES (GTT)

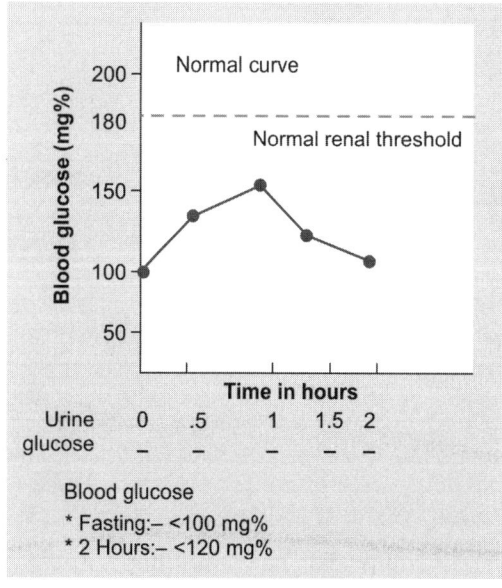

Fig.12.1: Normal curve.

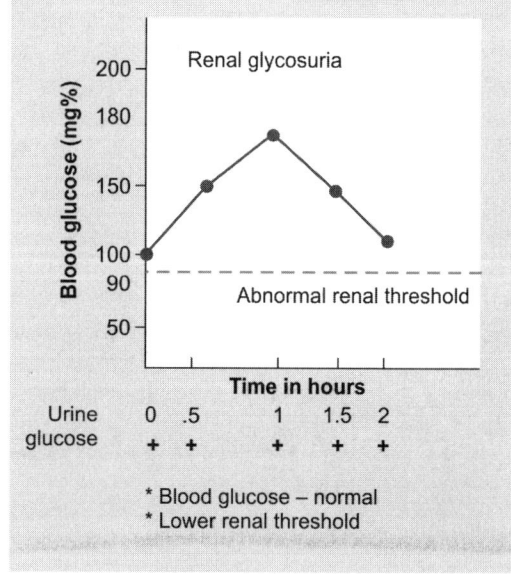

Fig.12.2: Renal glycosuria.

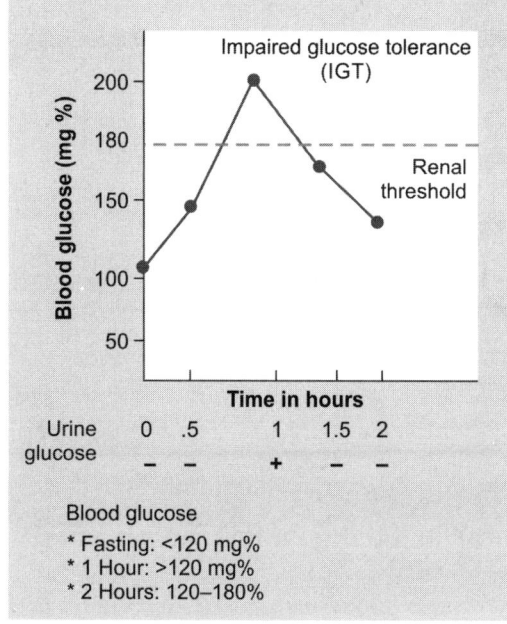

**Fig. 12.3:** Impaired glucose tolerance.

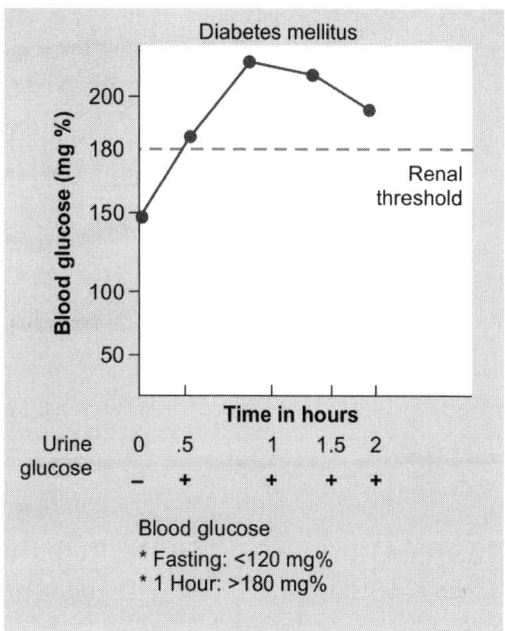

**Fig. 12.4:** Diabetes mellitus.

# CHAPTER 13

# Estimation of Serum and Urine Creatinine: Creatinine Clearance

**BI11.7** Demonstrate the estimation of serum creatinine and creatinine clearance.
**BI11.22** Calculate albumin: Globulin (AG) ratio and creatinine clearance.

## ESTIMATION OF CREATININE IN SERUM (BY ALKALINE PICRATE METHOD—BASED ON JAFFE'S REACTION)

### A. By Alkaline Picrate Method—Based on Jaffe's Reaction

Creatinine reacts with alkaline picrate reagent to form a reddish orange colored complex known as Creatinine Picrate. This color is measured in colorimeter at 540 nm using green filter. The intensity of the color is directly proportional to the concentration of creatinine present in the sample.

### Reagents

1. 10%     Sodium tungstate
2. 2/3 N   Sulfuric acid
3. 0.75 N  Sodium hydroxide
4. 0.04 M  Picric acid
5. Creatinine standard:
    a. Stock standard: 100 mg% (100 mg in 100 mL of N/10 HCl)
    b. Working standard: 4 mg% (4 mL of stock diluted to 100 mL).

### Procedure

#### A. Preparation of Protein-free Filtrate

Take 3 centrifuge tubes and label them as Blank (B), Test (T) and Standard (S) and proceed as follows:

| Reagents | Blank (B) | Standard (S) | Test (T) |
|---|---|---|---|
| Distilled water | 4 mL | 3.5 mL | 3.5 mL |
| Serum | — | — | 0.5 mL |
| Working standard | — | 0.5 mL | — |
| 10% Sodium tungstate | 0.5 mL | 0.5 mL | 0.5 mL |
| 2/3 N Sulfuric acid | 0.5 mL | 0.5 mL | 0.5 mL |
| Mix well. Wait for 10 minutes. Centrifuge the tube labeled T. | | | |

## B. Development of Color (Creatinine Picrate)

Take 3 long test tubes and label them as Blank (B), Standard (S) and Test (T).

To the tube labeled standard (S), pipette out 3 mL of diluted working standard solution from the centrifuge tube labeled (S). To the tube (T) pipette out 3 mL of protein-free filtrate from the centrifuge tube labeled (T). To the blank tube (B), pipette out 3 mL of solution from the centrifuge tube labeled (B). Arrange the 3 tubes in a rack, and add 1 mL of picric acid and 1 mL of 0.75 N NaOH to all the tubes. Mix well. Wait for 10 minutes at room temperature. Take reading in colorimeter at 540 nm using green filter.

| Reagents | Blank (B) mL | Standard (S) mL | Test (T) mL |
|---|---|---|---|
| Filtrate (Blank) | 3 | — | — |
| Filtrate (S) | — | 3 | — |
| Filtrate (T) | — | — | 3 |
| Picric acid | 1 | 1 | 1 |
| 0.75N NaOH | 1 | 1 | 1 |

### Calculation

Concentration of creatinine in 100 mL of serum

$$= \frac{ODT - ODB}{ODS - ODB} \times \frac{\text{Concentration of Std}}{\text{Actual Volume of Blood}} \times 100 \text{ mg}$$

$$= \frac{T-B}{S-B} \times \frac{0.012}{0.3} \times 100 \text{ mg}$$

$$= \frac{T-B}{S-B} \times \frac{12}{3} \text{ mg/dL}$$

$$= \frac{T-B}{S-B} \times 4 \text{ mg/dL}$$

### Conc. of Standard—Creatinine

- Stock standard Conc.: 100 mg%
- Working standard: 4 mg%
- 100 mL contains: 4 mg%
- Hence, 0.5 mL of standard contains: 0.02 mg%
- Total amount of filtrate: 5.0 mL
- 5.0 mL of filtrate contains: 0.02 mg
- Hence, 3 mL of filtrate contains: 0.02 × 3/5 = 0.06/5 = 0.012 mg.

## Actual Volume of Blood

- Actual volume of blood taken: 0.5 mL
- 5.0 mL of filtrate is from: 0.5 mL blood
- Hence, 3 mL of filtrate contains: 0.5 × 3/5 = 0.3 mL blood

$$\frac{\text{Conc. of Standard}}{\text{Actual Volume of Blood}} \times 100 = \frac{0.012}{0.3} \times 100 = \frac{1.2}{0.3} = 4$$

**Result:** Creatinine present in 100 mL of serum/plasma = ...mg %

# ESTIMATION OF CREATININE (USING PROTEIN-FREE FILTRATE) (BY ALKALINE PICRATE METHOD—BASED ON JAFFE'S METHOD)

## Principle

Creatinine reacts with alkaline picrate reagent to form a reddish orange colored complex known as creatinine picrate. This color is measured in colorimeter at 540 nm - green filter. The intensity of the color is directly proportional to the concentration of creatinine present in the sample.

## Reagents

1. Protein-free filtrate
2. 0.75 N sodium hydroxide
3. Standard picric acid
4. Stock standard: 100 mg% in N/10 HCl
5. Working standard: 4 mg% (4 mL of stock diluted to 100 mL with N/10 HCl).

## Procedure

Take three long test tubes. Mark them as Blank (B), Standard (S) and Test (T)

| Reagents | Blank (B) | Standard (S) | Test (T) |
|---|---|---|---|
| Distilled water | 3.0 | — | — |
| Protein-free filtrate | — | — | 3.0 |
| Working standard | — | 3.0 | — |
| Saturated picric acid | 1.0 | 1.0 | 1.0 |
| 0.75 N NaOH | 1.0 | 1.0 | 1.0 |

## Calculation

Concentration of creatinine in 100 mL of the given sample

$$= \frac{OD(T) - OD(B)}{OD(S) - OD(B)} \times 4 \text{ mg/dL}$$

$$= \frac{T - B}{S - B} \times 4 \text{ mg\%}$$

**Notes:**
Normal level of creatinine
Serum/Plasma: 0.6–1.2 mg/100 mL
Urine: 1.0–2.0 g/24 hrs

$$\begin{array}{cc}
\text{NH} \quad CH_3 & \text{NH} \quad NH_3 \\
\| \quad | & \| \quad | \\
C - N - CH_2 & C - N - CH_2 \\
| \quad | & | \quad | \\
NH - - CO & NH_2 \quad COOH \\
\text{Creatinine} & \text{Creatine}
\end{array}$$

Creatinine is the anhydride of creatine. Creatine is synthesized from 3 amino acids namely glycine, arginine and methionine. This occurs in 3 sites such as kidney, liver and skeletal muscles **(Fig. 13.1)**.

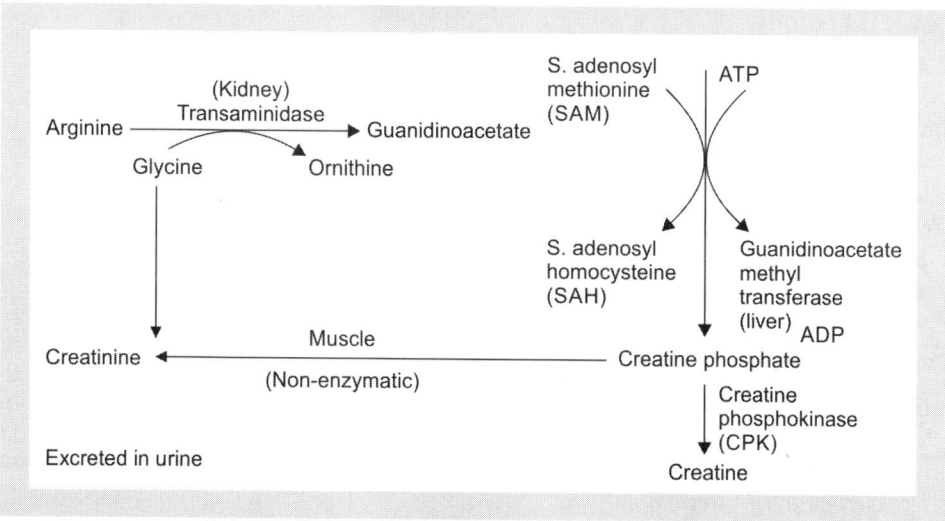

**Fig. 13.1:** Synthesis of creatinine.

Creatine phosphate (phosphagen) is the stored form of energy in muscle. About 2% of body creatine is daily excreted in urine as creatinine which is about 1–2 g/day for adults.

## Creatinine Clearance

This is the most sensitive method of assessing glomerular function. Creatinine is filtered fully by the glomerulus but partially reabsorbed by the tubules of the kidney.

$$\text{Creatinine clearance} = \frac{U \times V}{P}$$

U = Concentration of creatinine in urine (mg/100 mL)
P = Plasma creatinine concentration (mg/100 mL)
V = Urine flow in one minute (mL/min)

Normal level:
- Males: 85–125 mL/min.
- Females: 80–115 mL/min

## Clinical Interpretation

Increased level of creatinine in plasma is found in:
1. Renal diseases.
2. Congestive heart failure.
3. Obstruction of urinary tract.

Decreased creatinine clearance is a sensitive indicator of reduced glomerular filtration rate.

## Other Methods of Estimation of Creatinine

By using Lloyd's reagent-hydrated aluminium silicate: *Corynebacterium ureafaciens* (NC-Bacteria) removes creatine and then Lloyd's reagent is used to absorb the creatinine and alkaline picrate is then added to produce the color.

## Relevant Questions

1. What is creatinine?
2. What is the relationship between creatine and creatinine?
3. How is creatinine synthesized?
4. Where is creatinine synthesized?
5. What is the normal serum creatinine level?
6. How much of creatinine is excreted normally in urine per day?
7. Name the conditions in which creatinine levels will be increased?
8. What is creatinine clearance? What is its normal value?

## ■ CREATININE IN URINE AND CREATININE CLEARANCE

Creatinine is one of the normal constituents of urine. Daily excretion of creatinine in urine ranges from 1 to 2 g. On a normal diet, almost all the creatinine in the urine is endogenous. It is derived from muscle creatine and is the anhydride of creatine.
It is increased in fever and myopathy.

## Estimation of Creatinine in Urine (Jaffe's Reaction)

**Principle:** Creatinine in urine reacts with picric acid in the presence of sodium hydroxide to give an orange color (Jaffe's reaction). The color is measured at 500 nm.

**Method:** Dilute 1.0 mL urine to 100 mL with water in a standard flask. Therefore 5 mL of the diluted urine contains 0.05 mL urine.
  Mark three test tubes Standard (S), Test (T) and Blank (B). Proceed as follows:

| Reagent | Std (mL) | Test (mL) | Blank (mL) |
|---|---|---|---|
| Creatinine Working std | 5.0 | — | — |
| Diluted urine | — | 5.0 | — |
| Distilled water | — | — | 5.0 |

Add to each tube, 1 mL of 1% picric acid followed by 1.0 mL of 0.75 N NaOH, mixing after each addition. Stand for 15 minutes for color development. Set blank to 0 in a photometer at 500 nm (Yellow green filter). Read OD of the blank, standard and test.

## Calculations

$$\text{Creatinine in 0.05 mL urine} = \frac{ODT - ODB}{ODS - ODB} \times 0.05 \text{ mg}$$

$$\text{Creatinine in 100 mL urine} = \frac{ODT - ODB}{ODS - ODB} \times \frac{0.05}{0.05} \times 100 \text{ mg}$$

$$= \frac{ODT - ODB}{ODS - ODB} \times 100 \text{ mg}$$

## Creatinine Clearance

This is the most sensitive method of assessing glomerular function. Creatinine is filtered fully by the glomerulus but partially reabsorbed by the tubules of the kidney. It is defined as the number of mL of plasma cleared of creatinine per minute by the kidney.

$$\text{Creatinine clearance} = \frac{U \times V}{P}$$

U = Concentration of creatinine in urine (mg/100 mL)
P = Plasma creatinine concentration  (mg/100 mL)
V = Urine flow in 1 minute  (mL/min)

**Normal level:**
Males: 85–125 mL/min.
Females: 80–115 mL/min.

# CHAPTER 14

# Estimation of Urea

| | |
|---|---|
| BI11.21 | Demonstrate estimation of glucose, creatinine, urea and total protein in serum. |
| BI11.17 | Explain the basis and rationale of biochemical tests done in the following conditions:<br>• Diabetes mellitus<br>• Dyslipidemia<br>• Myocardial infarction<br>• Renal failure, gout<br>• Proteinuria<br>• Nephrotic syndrome<br>• Edema<br>• Jaundice<br>• Liver diseases, pancreatitis<br>• Acid-base disorders<br>• Thyroid disorders. |

## STRUCTURE OF UREA

$$\begin{array}{c} NH_2 \\ | \\ C=O \\ | \\ NH_2 \end{array}$$

Urea is the end product of protein metabolism in our body. Synthesis of urea occurs in the liver cells from ammonia and $CO_2$, which are the catabolic end products of amino acids.

## Methods of Estimation

- **Urease methods:** Using soya beans or horse gram powder, which contain urease. Urease acts on urea to liberate ammonia.
  a. Urease nesslerization method—Here ammonia is measured colorimetrically.
  b. Phenol-hypochlorite method using Berthelot reaction.
- **Direct colorimetric method:** Diacetyl monoxime method (DAM).
- **Stick tests (Ayostix).**
- **Autoanalyzer method.**

## A-1. Diacetyl Monoxime Method

**Principle:** Urea reacts with Diacetyl monoxime (DAM) in hot acid medium in the presence of ferric chloride and thiosemicarbazide to give a pink colored complex. The intensity of the color is directly proportional to the concentration of urea in the sample.

### Reagents

1. 10% Sodium tungstate
2. 2/3 N Sulfuric acid
3. Diacetyl monoxime/Thiosemicarbazide (DAM/TSC) reagent
4. Acid reagent (Mixture of orthophosphoric acid, Sulfuric acid and ferric chloride)
5. Urea standard:
   - Stock solution 1 g%
   - Working standard 50 mg%
   (5 mL of stock solution made up to 100 mL with DW).

### Procedure

### Preparation of Protein-free Filtrate

Take 3 centrifuge tubes and label them as Blank (B), Standard (S), and Test (T) and add reagents as given in the tabular column.

| Reagents | Blank (B) mL | Standard (S) mL | Test (T) mL |
| --- | --- | --- | --- |
| Distilled water | 3.6 | 3.4 | 3.4 |
| Blood Sample | — | — | 0.2 |
| Working standard | — | 0.2 | — |
| 10% Sodium Tungstate | 0.2 | 0.2 | 0.2 |
| 2/3N $H_2SO_4$ | 0.2 | 0.2 | 0.2 |
| Total | 4 | 4 | 4 |

Mix well and keep aside for 5 minutes. Centrifuge the tubes to get clear protein free filtrate. Take 3 test tubes and name them as Blank (B), Standard (S) and Test (T) and proceed as follows:

| Reagents | Blank (B) mL | Standard (S) mL | Test (T) mL |
| --- | --- | --- | --- |
| Protein free filtrate | 2.0 | 2.0 | 2.0 |
| DAM/TSC reagent | 3.0 | 3.0 | 3.0 |
| Acid reagent | 3.0 | 3.0 | 3.0 |

Mix well and keep the tubes in boiling water bath for exactly 20 minutes. Remove them afterwards and cool. Take readings at 540 nm (green filter).

## Calculation

Concentration of urea in mg/100 mL of serum

$$= \frac{\text{OD Test} - \text{OD Blank}}{\text{OD Std} - \text{OD Blank}} \times \frac{\text{Conc. of Std. (0.05 mg)}}{\text{Vol. of Sample in the filtrate (0.1 mL)}}$$

$$= \frac{T - B}{S - B} \times 50 \text{ mg\%}$$

**Result:** Urea present in 100 mL of serum = ................mg/dL.
- Normal level of urea in blood: 15–40 mg/100 mL or 8–20 mg of Blood urea nitrogen (BUN)/100 mL.
- Normal excretion of Urea per day: 15–30 g.

## Conc. of Standard—Urea

- Stock standard Conc.: 1000 mg%
- Working standard: 50 mg%
- 100 mL contains: 50 mg%
- Hence, 0.2 mL of standard contains: 0.1 mg%
- Total amount of filtrate: 4.0 mL
- 4.0 mL of filtrate contains: 0.1 mg
- Hence, 1 mL of filtrate contains: 0.1 × 2/4 = 0.05 mg.

## Actual Volume of Blood

- Actual volume of blood taken: 0.2 mL
- 4.0 mL of filtrate is from: 0.2 mL blood
- Hence, 1 mL of filtrate contains: 0.2 × 1/4 = 0.05 mL blood

$$\frac{\text{Conc. of Standard}}{\text{Actual Volume of Blood}} \times 100 = \frac{0.05}{0.1} \times 100 = 50$$

# ESTIMATION OF UREA (BY DIACETYL MONOXIME METHOD) (USING PROTEIN-FREE FILTRATE)

## Principle

Urea reacts with Diacetyl monoxime (DAM) in hot acid medium in the presence of ferric chloride and thiosemicarbazide to give a pink colored complex. The intensity of the color is directly proportional to the concentration of urea in the sample.

## Reagents

1. Protein-free filtrate (Sample)
2. Diacetyl monoxime, Thiosemicarbazide (DAM/TSC) Reagent
3. Acid mixture—mixture of Orthophosphoric acid, Sulfuric acid and Ferric chloride
4. Stock standard—1 g of urea of 100 mL of distilled water
5. Working standard—5 mL of stock diluted to 100 mL of distilled water (50 mg%).

## Procedure

Take three long test tubes. Mark them as Blank (B), Standard (S) and Test (T). Perform the test as follows:

| Reagents | Blank (B) mL | Standard (S) mL | Test (T) mL |
|---|---|---|---|
| Distilled water | 2.0 | — | — |
| Protein-free filtrate (sample) | — | — | 2.0 |
| Working standard | — | 2.0 | — |
| DAM/TSC reagent | 3.0 | 3.0 | 3.0 |
| Acid mixture | 3.0 | 3.0 | 3.0 |

Mix well and keep the test tubes in boiling water bath for exactly 20 minutes. Remove them afterwards and cool. Take readings at 540 nm (green filter).

## Calculation

Concentration of urea in mg/100 mL of the sample

$$= \frac{T-B}{S-B} \times 50 \text{ mg}$$

## Clinical Interpretation

**A. Increase in blood urea (uremia):** Occurs mainly in kidney diseases. This may be due to prerenal, renal and postrenal causes.
1. **Prerenal causes** (Blood flow to the kidneys is decreased)
   1. Dehydration as a result of salt and water depletion—mainly in vomiting and diarrhea
   2. Hematemesis, hemorrhage
   3. Shock—due to burns
   4. Cardiac failure.
2. **Renal causes** (all types of kidney diseases)
   1. Acute glomerulonephritis (AGN)
   2. Renal failure
   3. Malignant hypertension
   4. Congenital cystic kidney diseases.
3. **Postrenal causes** (due to obstruction to the flow of urine—causing urinary stasis)
   1. Enlarged prostate
   2. Stones in the urinary tract
   3. Stricture urethra
   4. Tumors of urinary bladder.

**B. Decrease in blood urea**
1. Low protein diet
2. Severe liver diseases
3. Overhydration-hemodilution.

**Normal daily urea excretion in urine:** 15–30 grams per day.
Decreased level of urea in urine found in acute renal insufficiency.
Increased level of urea in urine is found in prerenal causes, e.g., massive GI bleeding.

Urinary urea excretion is helpful in management of cases of acute renal failure and in assessing the ability of a transplanted kidney to handle an increasing dietary protein intake.

**Urea clearance:** It is the number of mL of blood, which contains the urea excreted in a minute by the kidneys.

$$\text{Urea clearance} = \frac{\text{mg. Urea excreted per minute}}{\text{mg. Urea per mL of blood/plasma}}$$

$$= \frac{UV}{B} \text{ or } \frac{UV}{P}$$

U = Urea in mg per 100 mL of urine
V = Volume of urine excreted per minute
B/P = mg urea per 100 mL of blood/plasma

### Normal range

- *Maximum clearance:* 60–95 mL/min (average 75)
- *Standard clearance:* 40–65 mL/min (average 54).

## Interpretations

- Increased level of urea clearance found in: early stages of nephrotic syndrome.
- Decreased level of urea clearance found in: Severe renal failure—below 20%.
- Uremic coma—below 5%.

Measurement of clearance is a test of glomerular filtration rate (GFR). Urea is filtered at the glomerulus fully and it is then partially (40%) reabsorbed by the tubules.

## Relevant Questions

1. What is the normal level of urea in blood and daily urine?
2. In which conditions urea level will be increased in blood?
3. How is urea synthesized? Where is it synthesized?
4. In which condition urea level will be decreased in blood?
5. What is urea clearance?
6. What are the methods by which urea can be estimated in blood?
7. What is DAM?
8. What is the principle of DAM method?

# CHAPTER 15

# Serum Proteins—Albumin: Globulin Ratio

**BI11.8** Demonstrate estimation of serum proteins, albumin and AG ratio.
**BI11.22** Calculate Albumin: Globulin (AG) ratio and creatinine clearance.

## ESTIMATION OF SERUM TOTAL PROTEINS, ALBUMIN: GLOBULIN (A:G) RATIO

Serum is a straw colored fluid separated when the blood has clotted and it lacks the clotting factors such as prothrombin and fibrinogen.

Plasma is the supernatant obtained when an anticoagulant added blood is centrifuged. It contains all the coagulation factors along with other proteins. Plasma contains hundreds of different proteins.

## Normal Values

- Total plasma proteins: 6.0–8.0 g/100 mL
- Albumin: 3.5–5.0 g/100 mL
- Globulins: 2.5–3.5 g/100 mL
- Fibrinogen: 200–400 mg/100 mL
- Albumin: Globulin ratio: 1.5 : 1.

All the plasma proteins are synthesized in liver except immunoglobulins which are synthesized in the plasma cells.

## Methods of Fractionation of Plasma Proteins

1. Half saturation with ammonium sulfate.
2. Cohn's fractionation by precipitating protein at different pH and ethyl alcohol gradient.
3. Electrophoresis.
4. Ultracentrifugation.

## Methods of Estimation of Plasma Proteins

1. Kjeldahl-Nesslerization method—by estimating nitrogen.
2. Lowery's method—estimation of Tyrosine in protein.
3. Copper sulfate specific gravity method.
4. Biuret method—commonly used method (Manual and autoanalyzer).

# Estimation of Serum Plasma Proteins by Biuret Method

## Principle

Substances which contain two $CO-NH_2$ groups join together directly or through a carbon or nitrogen atom and those which contain two or more peptide linkages give a blue to purple colored compound with alkaline copper solution. The reaction takes its name from the fact that the simple substance Biuret ($NH_2CONH\ CONH_2$) gives the same kind of color with cupric ions in alkaline medium. The intensity of the color is directly proportional to the concentration of total proteins present in the sample.

## Reagents

a. Biuret reagent (Sodium potassium tartrate, Sodium hydroxide, Copper sulfate and Potassium iodide).
b. Standard- Human albumin 8 g%

> 100 mL of Standard contains 8 g
> 
> 0.1 mL of Standard contains 0.008 g

## Procedure

Three test tubes are taken and named Blank, Standard and Test and proceeded as follows.

| Reagent | Blank (mL) | Standard (mL) | Test (mL) |
| --- | --- | --- | --- |
| Biuret reagent | 5.0 | 5.0 | 5.0 |
| Distilled water | 0.1 | — | — |
| Standard | — | 0.1 | — |
| Sample | — | — | 0.1 |

After mixing well, all the 3 test tubes are incubated for 20 minutes at room temperature and then the optical density is measured at 540 nm (green filter).

## Calculation

Concentration of total proteins
In the given serum

$$= \frac{T-B}{S-B} \times 8 \text{ g\%}$$

**Result:** Total protein present in 100 mL of serum/plasma is ............grams.

## Estimation of Serum Albumin

Albumin in serum/plasma is estimated by:
a. **BCG (Bromocresol green) method:** At pH 4.1 albumin acts as a cation and has binding affinity towards ionized BCG. At this pH albumin binds with BCG to form a blue colored complex which is measured at 620 nm.

*Reagents*
1. BCG dye in succinate buffer
2. Albumin standard
3. Normal saline—0.9% NaCl.

*Procedure*
First serum is diluted with saline (0.2 mL of serum diluted to 2.0 mL with saline). 3 test tubes are taken and labeled Blank (B), Standard (S) and Test (T) and proceeded as follows:

| Reagent | Blank (B) | Test (T) | Standard (S) |
|---|---|---|---|
| Normal Saline | 0.2 mL | | |
| Diluted Serum | | 0.2 mL | |
| Standard | | | 0.2 mL |
| BCG Dye | 5.0 mL | 5.0 mL | 5.0 mL |

All are mixed thoroughly and readings are taken at 620 nm after 10 minutes
Concentration of albumin (g%) = T/S × Amount of Std/Quantity of test × 1/10
Concentration of globulin = Total proteins—Albumin g%

b. **Reinhold's Biuret method:** In this method, globulin is precipitated by using 28% sodium sulfite. Then the albumin present in globulin free filtrate is measured by Biuret method (similar to estimation of total protein) by adding copper sulfate in alkaline medium to get a purple or violet color.

## Clinical Interpretation

Plasma protein level increased in:
1. Hemoconcentration: Due to dehydration from loss of fluids (vomiting and diarrhea)
2. Physiological causes: Standing position
   : Vigorous exercise
   : Excessive stasis while taking blood
3. Pathological causes
   a. Infective diseases: Tuberculosis
   b. Multiple myeloma

**Levels decreased in**
1. Malnutrition (Kwashiorkor)   : Physiological – pregnancy
2. Cirrhosis of liver            : Impaired intake
3. Malabsorption                 : Reduced synthesis
4. Excessive loss in urine       : Carcinoma stomach, peptic ulcer, enteritis, steatorrhea
5. Excessive loss from intestine : Nephrotic syndrome (proteinuria/albuminuria)
6. Loss from the skin            : Protein losing enteropathy
7. Severe hemorrhage             : Severe burns
8. Fever and after injury        : Increased catabolism

**Albumin: Globulin ratio (A:G ratio) = A/G**
Normal A:G ratio = 1.5–2.5
Reversal of A:G ratio:
- Reduction of albumin : Liver diseases
  : Nephrotic syndrome
- Elevation of globulin : Chronic infections

## Relevant Questions

1. What is the normal value of total proteins?
2. What are the normal values of albumin and globulin?
3. What is A:G ratio? What is its significance? What is the normal value?
4. What are plasma proteins? Name them.
5. What are the functions of plasma proteins?
6. How do you separate plasma proteins in the laboratory?
7. In which condition plasma proteins level will be (a) increased (b) decreased?
8. What is reversal of A:G ratio?
9. What is plasma?
10. What is serum?
11. What is the difference between plasma and serum?
12. By which method protein is estimated?
13. What is the principle of Biuret method?
14. What is Biuret?
15. Name the methods by which plasma protein level will be estimated in the laboratory?

# CHAPTER 16

# Serum Total Cholesterol

**BI11.9** Demonstrate estimation of serum cholesterol and HDL cholesterol.

## ■ ESTIMATION OF TOTAL CHOLESTEROL IN SERUM

Cholesterol occurs in blood in free and ester forms.

## Methods of Estimation of Cholesterol

1. Colorimetric methods using strong acid solvents.
2. Enzymatic assays.
3. Automated methods.

### *Colorimetric Method of Estimation of Total Cholesterol (Zak's Method)*

### Principle

Cholesterol reacts with ferric chloride in acetic acid and sulfuric acid to give reddish color which is measured colorimetrically.

### Reagents

1. Stock Ferric chloride reagent
2. Working Ferric chloride reagent—0.05%
3. Conc. Sulfuric acid
4. Cholesterol standard 200 mg%.

### Procedure

Arrange three big test tubes and mark them as B (Blank), S (Standard) and T (Test) and proceed as follows.

| Reagent | Blank (B) mL | Standard(S) mL | Test (T) mL |
|---|---|---|---|
| Standard Cholesterol 200 mg/dL | — | 0.1 | — |
| Serum or plasma | — | — | 0.1 |
| Working Ferric chloride | 10 | 9.9 | 9.9 |

All the reagents are mixed well by stirring with glass rod vigorously to enhance quick precipitation of the proteins in the test tube and centrifuged.

| Reagent | Blank (B) mL | Standard (S) mL | Test (T) mL |
|---|---|---|---|
| Supernatant | 5 | 5 | 5 |
| Conc. Sulfuric acid | 3 | 3 | 3 |

Mix well and let stand, for cooling about 15 minutes; take reading at 540 nm or green filter.

## Calculations

Concentration of cholesterol in mg/100 mL of serum

$$= \frac{\text{Test OD} - \text{Blank OD}}{\text{Std OD} - \text{Blank OD}} \times 200 \text{ mg/dL}$$

$$= \frac{\text{OD Test}}{\text{OD Test}} \times 200$$

*Note:*
12–14 hours fasting sample is preferable as it does not contain chylomicrons.
- Normal value of serum cholesterol—150–200 mg/dL.
- The value is increased physiologically with age, and also in pregnancy.

Abnormal increase in serum cholesterol (Hypercholesterolemia) is seen in:
- Nephrotic syndrome
- Diabetes mellitus—uncontrolled
- Atherosclerosis
- Obstructive jaundice
- Myxoedema
- Obesity
- Cirrhosis
- Xanthomatosis.

Decrease in cholesterol level (Hypocholesterolemia) is seen in:
- Hyperthyroidism
- Taking hypocholesterolemic drugs
- Pernicious anemia
- Hemolytic jaundice, liver diseases
- Malabsorption syndrome, malnutrition
- Oral contraceptive pills.

Normal ratio of free cholesterol and ester fraction—30% : 70%.

## Relevant Questions

1. What is normal blood cholesterol level?
2. How is cholesterol synthesized in human body?
3. Name the conditions in which cholesterol is high in blood.
4. In which conditions will there be hypocholesterolemia?
5. What is the ring of cholesterol called?
6. How many carbon atoms are there in cholesterol?

# CHAPTER 17

# Lipid Profile

**BI11.9** Demonstrate estimation of serum cholesterol and HDL cholesterol.
**BI11.10** Demonstrate the estimation of triglycerides.

## ESTIMATION OF HDL CHOLESTEROL AND TRIGLYCERIDES

### Plasma Lipid Profile

This includes the estimation of:
- Total Cholesterol
- High Density Cholesterol (HDL-C)
- Low Density Cholesterol (LDL-C)
- Triglycerides (Triacylglycerol–TAG).

**HDL-Cholesterol (HDL-C):** High Density Cholesterol-$\alpha$ Lipoprotein—It is also known as Good Cholesterol because it removes cholesterol from various tissues and transports it to the liver with the help of LCAT enzyme and Apo-A1.

**Principle of estimation:** LDL, VLDL and Chylomicrons are precipitated by treating the serum with phosphotungstic acid and magnesium chloride. The supernatant contains HDL which is obtained by centrifugation. This HDL is then measured by the same method (Zak's) for total cholesterol

**Normal value:** Men: 30–60 mg%; Women: 40–70 mg%
- Values increased in—Regular exercise and physical activity
- Values decreased in—malnutrition, lack of physical activity, Diabetes mellitus, Hypothyroidism and in liver diseases

**LDL-cholesterol (LDL-C):** Low Density Cholesterol-b Lipoprotein—It is also known as bad cholesterol because it delivers the cholesterol to peripheral tissues from liver. It increases the risk of coronary arterial disease (CAD) and atherosclerosis.

**Principle of estimation of LDL:** Estimation of LDL-C is a tedious process. So LDL is indirectly calculated from the serum Triacylglycerol by using Friedewald equation:

Total Cholesterol (Tc) = HDL-C+ LDL-C+ VLDL-C (mg%)
LDL-C = Tc – [HDL-C+ LDL-C] = Tc – [HDL-C+ TG/5]

**Normal levels of LDL—80–130 mg%**
LDL-C level is increased in—Coronary artery disease, Diabetes mellitus, Nephrotic syndrome, Cirrhosis of liver, Hypothyroidism, Obstructive jaundice.

## Triacylglycerols (TAG)/Triglycerides (TGL)

TAGs are present in Chylomicrons and in VLDL.

**Principles of estimation:** TAG is extracted from serum by propanol and saponified by propanolic potassium hydroxide to release glycerol, which is then oxidized by periodate to form formaldehyde. Then acetylacetone is added to formaldehyde to produce an yellow colored compound which is measured at 450 nm on a colorimeter.

Phospholipids present in the sample may interfere while estimating TAG. This is removed by adsorption on alumina.

### Reagents

Isopropanol, Alumina, Propanolic potassium hydroxide, Acetylacetone, sodium metaperiodate, TAG standard (200 mg/dL).

### Procedure

- 3 test tubes are taken and labeled Blank (B), Test (T) and Standard (S).

| Reagents | Blank (B) | Test (T) | Standard(S) |
|---|---|---|---|
| Distilled water | 0.2 mL | — | — |
| Standard | — | — | 0.2 mL |
| Serum | — | 0.2 mL | — |
| Isopropanol | 7.8 mL | 7.8 mL | 7.8 mL |
| Alumina | 1.0 g | 1.0 g | 1.0 g |

- All the contents are mixed thoroughly and centrifuged
- Another sets of 3 test tubes are taken and labeled Blank (B), Test (T) and Standard (S) and the steps are proceeded as follows:

| Reagents | Blank (B) | Test (T) | Standard (S) |
|---|---|---|---|
| Supernatant (from tube B) | 4.0 mL | — | — |
| Supernatant (from tube S) | — | Supernatant (from tube B) | 4.0 mL |
| Supernatant (from tube T) | — | 4.0 mL | — |
| Propanolic potassium hydroxide | 1.2 mL | 1.2 mL | 1.2 mL |
| Incubate at 65°C for 15 minutes | | | |
| Metaperiodate | 2.0 mL | 2.0 mL | 2.0 mL |
| Acetyl acetone | 1.0 mL | 1.0 mL | 1.0 mL |

- All the tubes are again incubated at 65°C for 30 minutes
- All the tubes are cooled and the OD readings of test and standard will be taken against blank at 450 nm (violet filter)

## Calculation

$$\text{Concentration of TAG} = \frac{\text{Test OD} - \text{Blank OD}}{\text{Std OD} - \text{Blank OD}} \times 200 \text{ mg/dL}$$

$$= \frac{\text{OD Test}}{\text{OD Std}} \times 200 \text{ mg\%}$$

## Interpretation
### Normal Value of Serum TAG is 50–200 mg/dL

Value increased in:
- Diabetes mellitus
- Alcoholism
- Hypothyroidism
- Chronic pancreatitis
- Lack of exercise.

Value decreased in:
- Malnutrition
- Hyperthyroidism.

# CHAPTER 18

# Serum Calcium and Phosphorus

**BI11.11** Demonstrate estimation of calcium and phosphorous.

## ESTIMATION OF SERUM CALCIUM

Human body contains 1–1.5 kg of calcium. Ninety-nine percent of this is present in bones and 1% in extra-cellular fluid.
- Normal blood calcium level is 9–11 mg/dL
- Different forms of calcium in plasma:
   a. Ionized calcium: 5 mg/dL
   b. Complexed with anions: 1 mg/dL
   c. Protein bound form: 4 mg/dL.

## Methods of Estimation of Total Calcium in Serum

- Using atomic absorption spectrophotometer
- Precipitation of calcium as calcium oxalate and liberation of oxalic acid by 1N Sulfuric acid followed by titration against standard potassium permanganate.

## Method of Clark and Collip of Estimation of Serum Calcium

### Principle

Total calcium present in serum is precipitated as calcium oxalate by adding ammonium sulfate solution. The calcium oxalate precipitate is washed with ammonia dissolved in acid and titrated at 70–80°C against standard permanganate. From the titer value calcium content of serum is calculated.

### Reagents:

- Ammonium oxalate (4 g/dL)
- 2% Ammonia solution (v/v)
- Potassium Permanganate solution—N/100 mL (0.01N)
- 1 N Sulfuric acid.

## Procedure

- 2 mL of serum and 2 mL of distilled water are taken in a centrifuge tube.
- Then 1 mL of saturated ammonium oxalate is added and mixed well and left undisturbed for 30 minutes.
- Calcium oxalate is precipitated after centrifuging.
- The clear supernatant is discarded.
- The precipitate is washed with 4 mL of dilute ammonia.
- Again the tube is centrifuged and the precipitate is washed again.
- Then 2 mL of 1.0N sulfuric acid is added and the tube is warmed at 80°C in water bath for 2 minutes.
- Titration of the solution is to be done with N/100 $KMnO_4$ to get a paie pink color.
- Blank is also titrated with 2 mL of 1.0N Sulfuric acid.

Total Calcium in the given sample = Titer value of test (T) - Blank (B) × 20 mg/dL.

## Interpretation

Normal blood calcium level is 9–11 mg/dL.

## Hypocalcemia

### Causes of Hypocalcemia

1. Deficiency of vitamin D—Rickets
2. Deficiency of Parathyroid hormone
3. Increased calcitonin—as in medullary carcinoma of thyroid
4. Deficiency of calcium
5. Increase in phosphorus level—as in renal failure and in renal tubular acidosis
6. Hypoalbuminemia.

### Symptoms of Hypocalcemia

1. Muscle cramps
2. Paresthesia in fingers
3. Neuromuscular irritability, twitching
4. Tetany (Chvostek's sign, Trousseau's sign)
5. Seizures
6. Bradycardia
7. Prolonged QT interval in ECG.

**Hypercalcemia:** Elevation in serum calcium level above 11mg/dL is known as hypercalcemia.

### Causes of Hypercalcemia

1. Hyperparathyroidism
2. Multiple myeloma
3. Paget's disease
4. Metastatic carcinoma of bone
5. Thyrotoxicosis

6. Benign familial hypercalcemia
7. Drugs—Thiazide diuretics, Excess Vit D, Lithium therapy.

## Symptoms of Hypercalcemia
1. Anorexia, nausea, vomiting
2. Polyuria, polydipsia
3. Renal stones
4. Ectopic calcification and pancreatitis
5. Blood alkaline phosphatase is increased.

## Relevant Questions
1. What is the normal value of serum calcium?
2. In which conditions it gets increased?
3. In which conditions calcium levels will be decreased?
4. Name the hormones that regulate calcium level?
5. What are the biochemical functions of calcium?
6. What is Tetany?
7. What are daily requirements of calcium?

# ■ ESTIMATION OF SERUM PHOSPHORUS (INORGANIC)

Total phosphorus in blood includes:
1. Inorganic phosphorus—Phosphates of alkali and earth metals—2–5 mg/100 mL
2. Organic or ester phosphorus—glycerophosphates—Nucleotide phosphates, etc. 15–30 mg/100 mL
3. Phospholipids—Lecithin, Cephalin, Sphingomyelin—10–16 mg/100 mL
4. Residual phosphorus—small amount—87% of phosphorus in the body is present in bones and the rest is present in cells and tissues.
5. Normal serum inorganic phosphorus is 2.5 to 4.5 mg per 100 mL in adults. In children the level is 4 to 7 mg per 100 mL.

The amount of phosphorus excreted in urine is about 1 g. This is in the form of inorganic phosphate only. Excretion depends upon the dietary phosphorus.

## Estimation of Phosphorus

### Method of Fiske and Subbarow

**Principle:** By the addition of iron trichloroacetic acid reagent, deproteinization is carried out. The supernatant is mixed with molybdic acid to form molybdic phosphate which is then reduced by $Fe^{++}$ to produce molybdenum blue. It is measured colorimetrically.

### Chemicals Required
1. Potassium dihydrogen phosphate ($KH_2PO_4$)
2. Ammonium molybdate
3. Trichloroacetic acid.
4. Thiourea

5. Ferrous ammonium sulfate ($6H_2O$)
6. Concentrated sulfuric acid.

## Reagents

1. Iron TCA reagent (stabilized)
2. Ammonium Molybdate (0.355 M)
3. Standard (phosphorus) 5 mg/100 mL.

Take 3 test tubes: Blank, Standard and Test. Take 5 mL of Iron TCA reagent in the test tubes labeled S and T. Add 0.2 mL of serum to tube T, 0.2 mL of standard to tube S and 5.2 mL of Iron TCA in tube B.

| Reagents | Test | Standard | Blank |
|---|---|---|---|
| Iron TCA | 5 mL | 5 mL | 5.2 mL |
| Standard | — | 0.2 mL | — |
| Serum | 0.2 mL | — | — |

Mix well. Filter through a Whatman No.1 filter paper. Add 0.5 mL Ammonium molybdate reagent to all the three tubes. Wait for 15 minutes. Color develops. Read at 620 nm (Red filter).

## Calculation

Concentration of phosphorus in the given sample of serum

$$= \frac{OD(T) - OD(B)}{OD(S) - OD(B)} \times \frac{\text{Concentration of Std}}{\text{Volume of Blood}} \times 100$$

$$= \frac{T-B}{S-B} \times \frac{0.01}{0.2} \times 100$$

$$= \frac{T-B}{S-B} \times \frac{10}{2}$$

$$= \frac{T-B}{S-B} \times 5 \, mg\%$$

## Result

The amount of phosphorus present in the given sample = ..................mg/100 mL

## Interpretation

**Increase** in serum Inorganic phosphorus (Hyperphosphatemia)
1. Chronic nephritis with renal failure.
2. Hypoparathyroidism.
3. Hypervitaminosis D.

**Decreased** serum Inorganic phosphorus (Hypophosphatemia)
1. Rickets, Osteomalacia—Vitamin D deficiency
2. Hyperparathyroidism
3. Disorder of renal tubular reabsorption—Fanconi syndrome.

Physiological fall of phosphorus occurs when there is increased carbohydrate utilization. Insulin therapy also has similar effect.

## Relevant Questions

1. What is the normal value of serum phosphorus?
2. In which conditions it gets increased?
3. In which conditions phosphorus level will be decreased?
4. Name the hormones that regulate phosphorus level?

# CHAPTER 19

# Serum Bilirubin

**BI11.12** Demonstrate the estimation of serum bilirubin.

## ■ ESTIMATION OF BILIRUBIN (DEMONSTRATION)

Bilirubin is the bile pigment formed from degradation of hemoglobin in the reticuloendothelial system. This bilirubin is then conjugated in the liver to form bilirubin glucuronides, which will be secreted in the bile and stored in gallbladder from where it passes into duodenum through common bile duct.

## Method of Malloy and Evelyn to Estimate Total and Direct Bilirubin

This method was based on Van den Bergh's reaction. Bilirubin is coupled with diazotized sulfanilic acid and converted to purple colored azobilirubin.

Conjugated bilirubin which is water soluble reacts fast with the Diazo reagent (Direct reaction). On the other hand, the free unconjugated bilirubin reacts slowly and requires an accelerator like methanol. Indirect reaction gives the value of total bilirubin.

### *Reagents*

1. Diazo reagent solution A : 100 mg of sulfanilic acid is dissolved in 1.5 mL of conc. HCl and made up to 100 mL with water.
   Solution B: 50 mg of sodium nitrite is dissolved in 100 mL of water.
   10 mL of solution A is mixed with 0.3 mL of solution B freshly every day before use.
2. Methanol.
3. 1.5% Hydrochloric acid.
4. Standard Bilirubin—10 mg of bilirubin is dissolved in 100 mL of chloroform (1 mL contains 0.1 mg).

### *Procedure*
### Estimation of direct and total bilirubin

The test tubes are labeled and proceeded as shown below:

|  | Total Bilirubin Total (T) mL | | Direct Bilirubin Direct (D) mL | | Standard STD (S) mL | |
|---|---|---|---|---|---|---|
|  | Test | Blank | Test | Blank | Std | Blank |
| Serum | 0.2 | 0.2 | 0.2 | 0.2 | — | — |
| Standard | — | — | — | — | 0.2 | — |
| Distilled water | 1.8 | 1.8 | 4.3 | 4.3 | 1.8 | 2.0 |
| Diazo reagent (A + B) | 0.5 | — | 0.5 | — | 0.5 | — |
| Diazo blank (A) | — | 0.5 | — | 0.5 | — | 0.5 |
| Methanol | 2.5 | 2.5 | — | — | 2.5 | 2.5 |

All the tubes are allowed to stand for 30 minutes and the optical densities are read in 540 nm using green filter.

## Calculations

Direct Bilirubin mg%

$$= \frac{OD\ of\ (D)\ Test - OD\ of\ (D)\ Blank}{OD(S) - OD(B)} \times \frac{Conc.\ of\ Std}{Vol.\ of\ Serum} \times 100$$

Total Bilirubin mg%

$$= \frac{OD(T)\ Test - OD(T)\ Blank}{OD\ of\ (S) - OD\ of\ (B)} \times \frac{Conc.\ of\ Std}{Vol.\ of\ Serum} \times 100$$

### Normal Value

Total serum Bilirubin = 0.2–1.2 mg/dL
Conjugated (Direct) Bilirubin = 0.1–0.4 mg/dL
Unconjugated (Indirect) Bilirubin = 0.2–0.7 mg/dL

## Interpretation

Hyperbilirubinemia of more than 2–3 mg/dL results in clinical jaundice.

### Classification of Jaundice

1. As per the nature of the bile pigment:
   a. Conjugated hyperbilirubinemia
   b. Unconjugated hyperbilirubinemia.
2. As per the site of lesion:
   a. Prehepatic
   b. Hepatic
   c. Posthepatic.
3. As per the pathological cause:
   a. Hemolytic
   b. Hepatocellular
   c. Obstruction to bile flow.

## Unconjugated hyperbilirubinemia (Hemolytic or Prehepatic)

**Causes:** Increased degradations of RBCs and hemolysis due to:
- Incompatible blood transfusion
- Rh incompatibility
- Hemolytic anemia.

## Conjugated hyperbilirubinemia (Hepatic and posthepatic)

- Hepatic jaundice—Viral hepatitis
- Posthepatic jaundice (Obstructive)
- Causes—Gallstones, Stricture in biliary tract
- Tumor pressing on bile duct—carcinoma of head of pancreas.

## Congenital hyperbilirubinemia

- Due to impaired glucuronyltransferase activity
  Crigler-Najjar syndrome, Gilbert's disease (Unconjugated)
- Defective biliary transport—Dubin Johnson's syndrome (Conjugated).

## Mixed hyperbilirubinemia

Both unconjugated and conjugated bilirubin are increased—due to hepatitis, drugs, poisoning and alcoholism.

# CHAPTER 20

# Serum Transaminases

**BI11.13** Demonstrate the estimation of SGOT/SGPT.

## ESTIMATION OF SERUM TRANSAMINASES (SGOT AND SGPT) (BY REITMAN AND FRANKEL METHOD)

- Serum glutamate oxaloacetate transaminase—SGOT (aspartate transaminase—AST)
- Serum glutamate pyruvate transaminase—SGPT (alanine transaminase—ALT)
- Transaminases are a group of enzymes which catalyze a reversible reaction in which there is the exchange of the alpha amino group between one alpha amino acid and another alpha keto acid forming a new alpha amino acid (II) and a new keto acid (II). Pyridoxal phosphate (PLP) is its coenzyme
- Aspartate + α-ketoglutarate $\xrightarrow{\text{SGOT/AST}}$ Oxaloacetate + Glutamate

- Alanine + α-ketoglutarate $\xrightarrow{\text{SGPT/AST}}$ Pyruvate + Glutamate

## Principle

For AST: The serum is added to a buffered solution of α-ketoglutarate and aspartate and the resulting oxaloacetate formed after incubation is measured colorimetrically by reaction with dinitrophenylhydrazine (DNPH).

For ALT: The serum is added to a buffered solution of α-ketoglutarate and alanine and the resulting pyruvate formed after incubation is measured colorimetrically by reaction with dinitrophenylhydrazine (DNPH).

The absorbance of the brown colored dinitrophenylhydrazone is measured at 520 nm using green filter.

## Estimation of SGOT (AST)/SGPT (ALT)

### Reagents

1. AST or OT substrate for SGOT/ALT substrate for SGPT
2. Sodium pyruvate standard
3. DNPH—(2:4 Dinitrophenylhydrazine)
4. 0.4 N NaOH

**Procedure:** Take 4 clean and dry test tubes and mark them Test (T), Control (C), Standard (S) and Blank (B) Add 1.0 mL of substrate in all the tubes. Keep the test tubes in the incubator at 37°C for 3 minutes. Then add 0.2 mL of serum in the test (T) alone and continue the incubation for 60 minutes for AST and 30 minutes for ALT. After that take the test tubes out and add 1.0 mL of DNPH in all the tubes and 0.2 mL of serum in the control and wait for 20 minutes at room temperature. Then add 10.0 mL of 0.4 N NaOH in all the tubes. Wait for 10 minutes. Take readings at 520 nm.

*The same procedure should be followed for both AST and ALT—substrates are different.

## Procedure

| Reagents | Test | Control | Standard | Blank |
|---|---|---|---|---|
| Substrate | 1.0 mL | 1.0 mL | 1.0 mL | 1.0 mL |
| Serum | 0.2 mL | — | — | — |
| Standard | — | — | 0.2 mL | — |
| Dist.Water | — | — | — | 0.2 mL |
| Incubation at 37°C 30 minutes for AST/60 minutes for AST. | | | | |
| DNPH | 1.0 mL | 1.0 mL | 1.0 mL | 1.0 mL |
| Serum | — | 0.2 mL | — | — |
| Mix well and wait for 20 minutes at room temperature | | | | |
| 0.4 N NaOH | 10.0 mL | 10.0 mL | 10.0 mL | 10.0 mL |
| Wait for 5 minutes and take readings at 520 Nm. | | | | |

## Calculation

Concentration of AST = $\dfrac{T-C}{S-B} \times \dfrac{0.4}{0.2} \times \dfrac{1000}{60} \times 0.487$ IU/L

Concentration of ALT = $\dfrac{T-C}{S-B} \times \dfrac{0.4}{0.2} \times \dfrac{1000}{30} \times 0.487$ IU/L

## Result

The Concentration of SGOT/SGPT = ..........................IU/L.

## Interpretation

1. Aspartate aminotransferase (AST/SGOT)
   - Normal serum level of AST—8–40 U/L
   - In myocardial infarction AST level rises sharply and reaches a peak within 48 hours. It takes 4–5 days to return to normal level
   - It is also a marker of liver injury and its level is increased in hepatitis and in cancer of liver.
2. Alanine transaminase (ALT/SGPT)
   - Normal serum level of ALT—13–35 U/L for males and 10–35 U/L for females
   - It is highly increased in toxic or viral hepatitis and moderately increased in cirrhosis and chronic hepatitis.

# CHAPTER 21
# Serum Alkaline Phosphatase

**BI11.14** Demonstrate the estimation of alkaline phosphatase.

## ESTIMATION OF SERUM ALKALINE PHOSPHATASE (ALP)

Alkaline phosphatase has different isoforms such as alpha-1, alpha-2 heat labile, alpha-2 heat stable, pre beta, gamma leukocyte ALP, etc. Its optimum pH is 9–10. It is a Zinc containing enzyme activated by Magnesium and Manganese

1. Alpha-1 ALP – (10% of total)—synthesized by epithelial cells of biliary canaliculi. It is increased in obstructive jaundice and metastatic carcinoma of liver.
2. Alpha-2 heat labile ALP – (25% of total)—produced by hepatic cells. It is increased in hepatitis.
3. Alpha-2 heat stable ALP – (1% of total) placental origin and found in blood in normal pregnancy.
4. An isoenzyme which resembles – alpha-2 heat stable ALP, called Regan Isoenzyme (carcino-placental isoenzyme) is increased in carcinoma of lung, liver and gut and also in chronic smokers.
5. Pre beta ALP (50% of total) synthesized from bone. Increased in bone diseases.
6. Gamma ALP (10% of total): It is increased in ulcerative colitis.
   It is synthesized from the intestine.
7. Leukocyte alkaline phosphatase (LAP)—synthesized from leukocytes. It is increased in lymphomas and decreased in chronic myeloid leukemia.

## Determination of Alkaline Phosphatase (4-Amino Antipyrine Method)

**Principle:** Alkaline phosphatase hydrolyzes disodium phenylphosphate liberating phenol which is proportional to the enzyme activity. The phenol is reacted with 4-aminoantipyrine to give with alkaline ferricyanide, a reddish colored product which is measured at 510 nm.

## Procedure

Mark 4 tubes, Blank (B), Standard (S), Control(C) and Test (T). Proceed as follows:

| Reagents | B (mL) | S (mL) | T (mL) | C (mL) |
|---|---|---|---|---|
| Buffer | 1.1 | 1.1. | 1.0 | 1.0 |
| Substrate (Disodium phenyl phosphate) | — | — | 1.0 | 1.0 |
| Distilled water | 1.0 | — | — | — |
| Phenol working std | — | 1.0 | — | — |
| Serum | — | — | 0.1 | — |

Incubate at 37°C the tubes marked 'T' and 'C' for exactly 15 minutes.

| Reagents | B (mL) | S (mL) | T (mL) | C (mL) |
|---|---|---|---|---|
| NaOH (0.5 N) | 0.8 | 0.8 | 0.8 | 0.8 |
| Serum | — | — | — | 0.1 |
| Sodium Bicarbonate | 1.2 | 1.2 | 1.2 | 1.2 |
| Aminoantipyrine | 1.0 | 1.0 | 1.0 | 1.0 |
| Pot. Ferricyanide | 1.0 | 1.0 | 1.0 | 1.0 |

Mix well after each addition. The final color produced is measured at 510 nm or green filter.

## Calculation

$$= \frac{\text{OD Test} - \text{OD Control}}{\text{OD Std} - \text{OD Blank}} \times 10 \text{ KA Unit}$$

## Interpretation

- Normal serum value of ALP-3-13 KA units (King Armstrong Units) (40–125 U/L)
- Mild increase
  - Children (due to increased osteoblastic activity)
  - Normal pregnancy (increase in placental isoenzyme).
- High increase of ALP
  - Extrahepatic obstruction (cholestasis)
  - Bone diseases
  - Paget's disease
  - Rickets
  - Osteomalacia.

# CHAPTER 22

# Serum Uric Acid

**BI11.17** Explain the basis and rationale of biochemical tests done in renal failure, gout.

## ■ ESTIMATION OF URIC ACID IN SERUM

Uric acid is the end product of the metabolism of purines which are Adenine, Guanine, Xanthine and Hypoxanthine. Purines are present in the nucleic acids.

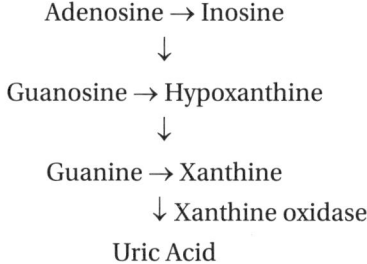

**Uric acid** is one of the non-protein nitrogenous substances. In the kidney, uric acid is fully filtered by the glomerulus but partially reabsorbed in the proximal convoluted tubules.

The normal uric acid level in blood
- **Males:** 3.5–7.0 mg/dL
- **Females:** 2.5–6.5 mg/dL

Daily urinary excretion of uric acid is 250–750 mg. At the body pH, uric acid exists usually as monosodium urate salt.

## Methods of Estimation of Uric Acid

1. **Method of Brown:** Using sodium cyanide and Phosphotungstic acid
2. **Method of Caraway:** Using sodium carbonate and Phosphotungstic acid.
3. **Uricase method.**

### A. Estimation of Serum Uric Acid (Method of Caraway)

**Principle:** Uric acid is oxidized to allantoin by phosphotungstic acid. This acid is further reduced to tungsten blue in alkaline sodium carbonate medium. The color of the solution is proportional to the concentration of uric acid present in the sample. It is measured in the photoelectric colorimeter at 620 nm (red filter).

## Reagents

a. 10% Sodium Tungstate
b. 2/3 N Sulfuric acid
c. Phosphotungstic acid.
d. 10% Sodium carbonate.
e. Standard uric acid solution (10 mg%)

## Procedure

Take 3 test tubes. Label them as Blank, Standard, Test and proceed as follows:

| Reagent | Blank (mL) | Standard (mL) | Test (mL) |
|---|---|---|---|
| Distilled water | 4.0 | 3.5 | 3.5 |
| Serum | — | — | 0.5 |
| Standard | — | 0.5 | — |
| 10% Sod. Tungstate | 0.5 | 0.5 | 0.5 |
| 2/3 N $H_2SO_4$ | 0.5 | 0.5 | 0.5 |

Mix well and centrifuge to get a clear filtrate. Take 3 test tubes. Name them as (B) Blank, (S) Standard and (T) Test.

| Reagent | Blank (mL) | Standard (mL) | Test (mL) |
|---|---|---|---|
| Filtrate | 2.5 | 2.5 | 2.5 |
| Sodium Carbonate | 1.0 | 1.0 | 1.0 |
| Let stand for 10 minutes and then add Phosphotungstic acid | 1.0 | 1.0 | 1.0 |

Mix well and take reading at 620 nm using red filter.

## Calculation

Conc. of uric acid in the given sample of serum

$$= \frac{OD(T) - OD(B)}{OD(S) - OD(B)} \times \frac{\text{Concentration of Std}}{\text{Actual volume of Blood}} \times 100$$

$$= \frac{OD(T) - OD(B)}{OD(S) - OD(B)} \times \frac{0.025}{0.25} \times 100$$

$$= \frac{T - B}{S - B} \times \frac{2.5}{0.25}$$

$$= \frac{T - B}{S - B} \times 10 \text{ mg\%}$$

## Result

Concentration of uric acid present in 100 mL of serum/Plasma is .........mg.

## Conc. of Standard—Uric Acid

- Stock standard Conc.: 100 mg%
- Working standard: 10 mg%

- 100 mL contains: 10 mg%
- Hence, 0.5 mL of standard contains: 0.05 mg%
- Total amount of Filtrate: 5.0 mL
- 5.0 mL of Filtrate contains: 0.05 mg
- Hence, 2.5 mL of Filtrate contains: $0.05 \times 2.5/5 = 0.025$ mg%.

### Actual Volume of Blood
- Actual volume of blood taken: 0.5 mL
- 5.0 mL of Filtrate is from: 0.5 mL blood
- Hence, 2.5 mL of Filtrate contains: $0.5 \times 2.5/5 = 0.25$ mL blood

$$\frac{\text{Conc. of Standard}}{\text{Actual Volume of Blood}} \times 100 = \frac{0.025}{0.25} \times 100 = 10$$

## B. Estimation of Uric Acid (Using Protein-free Filtrate) (Method of Caraway)

**Principle:** Uric acid is oxidized to allantoin by Phosphotungstic acid. This acid is further reduced to tungsten blue in alkaline sodium carbonate medium. The color of the solution is proportional to the concentration of uric acid present in the sample. It is measured in the photoelectric colorimeter at 620 nm (red filter).

### Reagents
- Protein-free filtrate
- Phosphotungstic acid
- 10% Sodium carbonate.
- Stock standard—100 mg %
- Working standard—5 mL diluted to 100 mL with distilled water (5 mg%)

### Procedure
Take 3 long test tubes. Mark them as Blank (B), Standard (S), Test (T).

| Reagent | Blank (mL) | Standard (mL) | Test (mL) |
|---|---|---|---|
| Distilled water | 2.5 | — | — |
| Protein-free filtrate | — | — | 2.5 |
| Working standard | — | 2.5 | — |
| 10% Sodium carbonate | 1.0 | 1.0 | 1.0 |
| Phosphotungstic acid | 1.0 | 1.0 | 1.0 |

Mix well and the reading is taken after 15 minutes at 620 nm in red filter.

### Calculation
Conc. of uric acid in the given sample

$$= \frac{OD(T) - OD(B)}{OD(S) - OD(B)} \times 5 \text{ mg\%}$$

## Clinical Interpretation

A  Increased uric acid level (Hyperuricemia) will be seen in
*Congenital*:
  i. Gout
  ii. Lesch-Nyhan syndrome – X-linked recessive disorder.

*Acquired*
  i. Renal diseases
  ii. Leukemia
  iii. Toxemia of pregnancy
  iv. After treatment of malignant tumors.
  v. Psoriasis.

**Gout:** When the increased level of uric acid exceeds the solubility limit, it results in crystallization of sodium urate in soft tissues and joints to form Tophi, causing the inflammatory condition – acute gouty arthritis which will progress to chronic gouty arthritis. The typical gouty arthritis affects the first metatarsophalangeal joint (Big toe) but all other joints may be affected. The joints are painful and the synovial fluid shows presence of birefringent monosodium urate crystals. Chronic gout may end in renal damage due to the deposition of sodium urate in the renal medulla.

Inherited Gout is caused due to the high activity of the enzyme Phosphoribosyl Pyrophosphate (PRPP) synthetase and due to the partial deficiency of the enzyme Hypoxanthine-guanine phosphoribosyltransferase (HGPRTase).

### C. Decreased Level of Uric Acid (Hypouricemia) is Seen in:

1. Wilson's disease
2. Fanconi syndrome
3. Immunodeficiency: Adenosine deaminase deficiency
4. Xanthinuria: Congenital deficiency of Xanthine oxidase

## Relevant Questions

1. What is uric acid?
2. How is uric acid formed?
3. What is the normal value of uric acid in blood?
4. What is the normal urinary excretion of uric acid per day?
5. In which diseases, does the uric acid level increase?
6. What is gout? What is it due to?
7. What is Tophi?
8. Give example for some hypouricemic condition.
9. By which method did you do the estimation?
10. What is the principle of Caraway method?

# SECTION 4

# Equipments and Procedures

## Section Outline

23. Point of Care Testing
24. pH Meter
25. Paper Chromatography and Thin Layer Chromatography
26. Protein Electrophoresis
27. Polyacrylamide Gel Electrophoresis
28. Electrolyte Analysis
29. Arterial Blood Gas Analyzer
30. Enzyme-linked Immunosorbent Assay
31. Immunodiffusion
32. Autoanalyzer
33. DNA Isolation from Blood/Tissues

# CHAPTER 23

# Point of Care Testing

| | |
|---|---|
| BI11.17 | Explain the basis and rationale of biochemical tests done in the following conditions:<br>• Diabetes mellitus<br>• Dyslipidemia<br>• Myocardial infarction<br>• Renal failure, gout<br>• Proteinuria<br>• Nephrotic syndrome<br>• Edema<br>• Jaundice<br>• Liver diseases, pancreatitis<br>• Acid-base disorders<br>• Thyroid disorders |
| BI11.19 | Outline the basic principles involved in the functioning of instruments commonly used in biochemistry laboratory and their applications. |

## ■ POINT OF CARE TESTING (POCT)

Point of care testing (POCT) includes the tests that are done outside the clinical laboratory but nearer to the bedside of the patient. This can be done by the patient himself—self testing or by any of the members of the family or any other qualified person in the hospital apart from the technicians like nurses, paramedics or doctors.

POCT can be done primarily at home, office, clinic, community care center, etc. Secondarily POCT can be done at emergency wards, ICU, operation theaters and outpatient departments and in ambulance services.

## Advantages

- Quick and early result
- Reduced turnaround time (TAT)
- Minimizing the delay in sample collection, transport, etc.
- Better patient care
- For prompt treatment to the patients by the physician.

## POCT Tests

- They may be based on instruments or non-instrument based like enzyme assays, immune assays, etc.
- A minute drop or a few microliter of sample is sufficient to do the test. Blood, serum, plasma, saliva, urine, CSF can be used as sample.
- Qualitative POCT—gives positive and negative readable endpoint results, e.g., Pregnancy test kit, urinary dipstick for albumin, glucose, etc.
- Semiquantitative POCTs—Urinary dipsticks.
- Instrument-based POCTs—Easy to operate, e.g., Home blood glucose monitoring, noninvasive pulse oximeter to find out the oxygen saturation of blood.
- This system involves disposable one-time consumables to be used hygienically.

## Urine Dipstick Test

- Based on dry chemistry system
- The test strips are made up of either plastic or paper.
- Paper strips are used for specific tests such as pH measurement, specific gravity, glucose, albumin, ketone bodies, etc.

## Estimation of Blood Glucose by Glucometer (Fig. 23.1)

- This is the most commonly used POCT for monitoring blood glucose by diabetic patients.
- POCT measures the glucose level in arterial capillary blood obtained from a fingertip.
- The strips consist of an enzyme-based assay system usually glucose oxidase method.
- The glucose level covers a wide range from low to high levels like 10 mg to 500 mg/dL. The required sample will be 0.5–1.0 µL. The results will be obtained within 5–10 seconds.

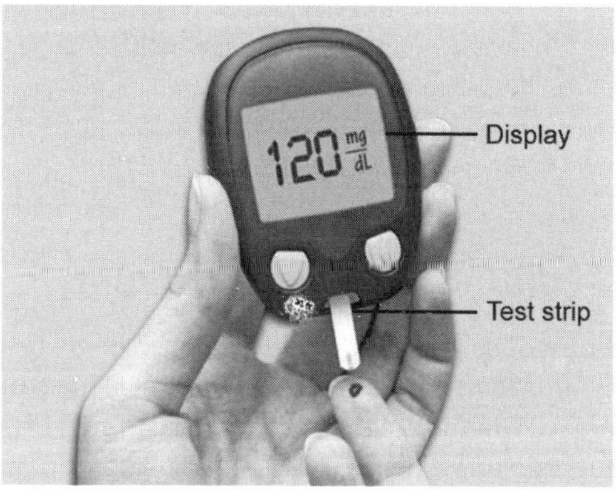

### Procedure

- The fingertip or the punctured site should be cleaned and dried
- The reagent strip is then inserted into the glucometer.
- The site is punctured with a lancet to get a good blood droplet
- The blood droplet is applied to the test strip and the reading is noted from the display in the glucometer.

**Fig. 23.1:** Glucometer.

# CHAPTER 24

# pH Meter

| BI11.16 | Observe use of commonly used equipment/techniques in biochemistry including:<br>• **pH meter**<br>• Paper chromatography of amino acid<br>• Protein electrophoresis<br>• TLC, PAGE<br>• Electrolyte analysis by ISE<br>• Autoanalyzer<br>• DNA isolation from blood/tissue |
|---|---|
| BI11.19 | Outline the basic principles involved in the functioning of instruments commonly used in biochemistry laboratory and their applications. |

## ■ pH METER (FIG. 24.1)

This apparatus is used to determine the pH of a solution more accurately by potential measurement of certain electrodes.

## Electrometric Determination of pH

### Principle

When a glass membrane that separates two different solutions having different pH, a potential difference is found to be present between the surfaces of the glass. The potential is measured against a standard calomel electrode.

### Parts of a pH Meter

1. Potentiometer
2. Reference Calomel Electrode—It has metallic mercury in contact with mercuric chloride in potassium chloride solution.

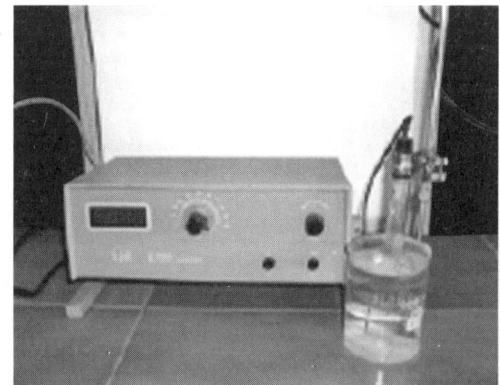

**Fig. 24.1:** pH meter.

3. Glass electrode—It is a bulb of special glass which is filled with some standard electrolytes such as 0.1N HCl in contact with a suitable metallic electrode.
4. Solution of known pH.

## Operation of a pH Meter

pH meter is turned 15 minutes prior to use and then it is calibrated with reference buffers. Then the electrodes are dipped in the test solution for 30 seconds and the reading is taken.

The glass electrodes should be carefully washed after each pH determination.

# CHAPTER 25
# Paper Chromatography and Thin Layer Chromatography

| | |
|---|---|
| BI11.16 | Observe use of commonly used equipment/techniques in biochemistry including:<br>• pH meter<br>• **Paper chromatography of amino acid**<br>• Protein electrophoresis<br>• **TLC**, PAGE<br>• Electrolyte analysis by ISE<br>• Autoanalyzer<br>• DNA isolation from blood/tissue. |
| BI11.19 | Outline the basic principles involved in the functioning of instruments commonly used in biochemistry laboratory and their applications. |
| BI11.5 | Describe the use of paper chromatography. |

## ■ PAPER CHROMATOGRAPHY (SEPARATION OF AMINO ACIDS)

Chromatography may be defined as a technique in which the components of mixture containing amino acids and many other physiologically important substances like carbohydrates, lipids are separated. In addition, this can be used:

1. To establish the identity of one or more substances in a mixture
2. To estimate the molecular mass of a compound
3. To concentrate solute molecules
4. To purify a substance of particular interest from other interfering compounds in a sample and
5. To aid in structure elucidation.

## Principle

It is based on the principle of partition of the compounds to be separated between a stationary phase and a moving phase. Stationary phase is the supporting filter paper holding the water molecules in its pores. Moving phase is the organic solvent contained in the solvent mixture. Migration is effected by the flow of the solvent which percolates through the stationary phase. Solute molecules are separated by one or other of the physicochemical processes such as surface adsorption, solvent partition, molecular sieving and ion exchange.

## Technique (Fig. 25.1)

Prepare the solvent mixture of butanol, acetic acid and water in the proportion of 24/6/10 mL and place it in a shallow trough and cover it with the bell jar for saturation of the chamber. Take a Whatman No. 1 filter paper of dimensions appropriate (14" × 12") for the chromatographic chamber (bell jar) used. Draw a line with a pencil along the width of the paper 5 cm from its edge. Mark points on the line 2 cm from the edge at distances of 2 cm. Apply the standard in the form of a small spot 4 or 5 times each time allowing the sample to dry perfectly (10 uL). The test sample is applied in the same manner but for more number of times in order to get a good separation. Fold the paper along the width holding the edges without touching the rest of the area and stitch the edges at 3 points. Place the folded paper in the trough containing the solvent mixture with the pencil line at the bottom. Close it with bell jar without touching the paper. The solvent moves up on the paper by capillary action, carrying with it the amino acids. The run is stopped after 18–20 hours. Mark the solvent front with a pencil. Remove the stitches and hold the paper using clips and air dry it. Spray it with ninhydrin stain 0.5% in acetone. Air dry the paper and keep it for 5 minutes in an oven maintained at 500°C. The amino acids appear as distinct purple spots. Calculate the Rf values for amino acids in the given mixture and identify them by comparing with the Rf values of known amino acids used as standard. Rf value is always less than one.

$$Rf = \frac{\text{Distance travelled by the solute (amino acid)}}{\text{Distance travelled by the solvent}}$$

Distance travelled by solute = Distance from the center of the spot applied to the center of the spot migrated.

Distance travelled by solvent = Distance from the pencil line to the marked solvent front.

## Clinical Significance

Normally, very low amounts of amino acids are present in the urine. In specific amino acid metabolic disorders classified as inborn errors of metabolism large amounts of specific amino acids or their metabolites are excreted in the urine which can be identified by this technique.

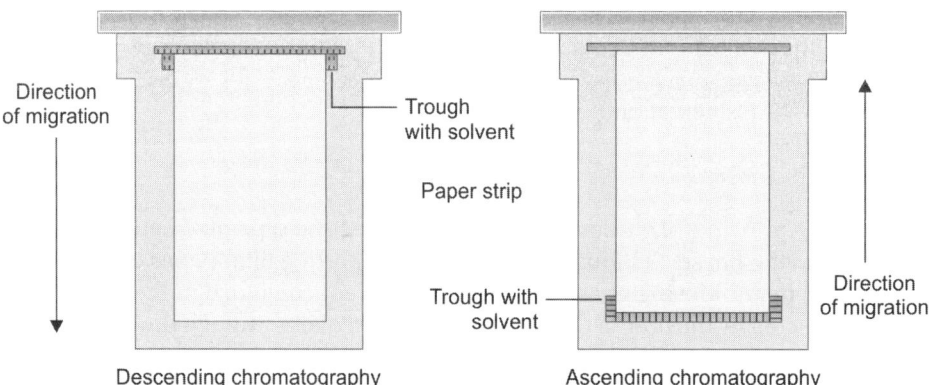

**Fig 25.1:** Paper chromatography.

# THIN LAYER CHROMATOGRAPHY (TLC)

- This is liquid-liquid chromatography under partition
- A TLC plate is a sheet of glass, metal, or plastic which is coated with a thin layer of a solid adsorbent (usually silica or alumina).
- A small amount of the mixture to be analyzed is spotted near the bottom of this plate. The TLC plate is then placed in a shallow pool of a solvent in a developing chamber so that only the very bottom of the plate is in the liquid. This liquid, or the eluent, is the mobile phase, and it slowly rises up the TLC plate by capillary action.
- As the solvent moves past the spot that was applied, the components in the mixture differ in solubility and in the strength of their adsorption to the adsorbent and some components will be carried further up the plate than others.
- When the solvent has reached the top of the plate, the plate is removed from the developing chamber, dried, and the separated components of the mixture are visualized.
- After the run is over, the paper or the plate is dried.
- Location reagents such as ninhydrin will be sprayed for aminoacids and proteins; sulphuric acid sprayed for phospholipids and diphenylamine for sugars.
- If the compounds are colored, visualization is straightforward. Usually the compounds are not colored, so a UV lamp is used to visualize the plates. (The plate itself contains a fluorescent dye which glows everywhere except where an organic compound is on the plate.)
- Spots are identified and the distance travelled by the solute and solvent are marked and Rf value calculated.

Rf value is the ratio of distance travelled by substance and the distance travelled by the solvent. It is a constant for a particular solvent system:

$$Rf = \frac{\text{Distance travelled by solvent front}}{\text{Distance travelled by substance}}$$

The Rf values are strongly dependent upon the nature of the adsorbent and solvent.

# CHAPTER 26
# Protein Electrophoresis

| BI11.16 | Observe use of commonly used equipment/techniques in biochemistry including:<br>• pH meter<br>• Paper chromatography of amino acid<br>• **Protein electrophoresis**<br>• TLC, PAGE<br>• Electrolyte analysis by ISE<br>• Autoanalyzer<br>• DNA isolation from blood/tissue. |
|---|---|
| BI11.19 | Outline the basic principles involved in the functioning of instruments commonly used in biochemistry laboratory and their applications. |

## ■ ELECTROPHORESIS

### Principle of Electrophoresis

- The term electrophoresis refers to the movement of charged particles through an electrolyte when subjected to an electric field.
- Cations (positively charged ions) move towards cathode and anions (negative) to anode.
- When a biological mixture is subjected to electrophoresis, the compounds in the mixture move in relation to their net charge, size, molecular weight and mass and get separated according to these characteristics, so that the desired compound can be identified and isolated.
- Types of electrophoresis:
  1. Zone electrophoresis (Paper, Gel)
  2. Isoelectric focussing
  3. Immunoelectrophoresis.

### Supporting Media Used in Electrophoresis

**Supporting medium** is the surface on which electrophoresis is carried out. It may be agar gel or agarose gel, cellulose acetate membrane, filter paper, polyacrylamide gel electrophoresis (PAGE).

## PAGE

Polyacrylamide gel electrophoresis (PAGE): This is a type of electrophoresis where the supporting medium is polyacrylamide gel. It has a molecular sieving effect that makes the separation efficient.

## ■ PAPER ELECTROPHORESIS (SEPARATION OF SERUM PROTEINS)

Electrophoresis refers to the migration of charged particles in an electric field. It is a valuable diagnostic tool in clinical laboratory. It is used for the separation of serum proteins, serum lipoproteins, isoenzymes, immunoglobulins, abnormal hemoglobin and many other compounds. Proteins are negatively charged when they are placed in a buffer alkaline to their isoelectric pH and move towards anode. They are positively charged when placed in a buffer acidic to their isoelectric pH and move towards cathode. The rate of migration of particles depends upon the number of charges each carries and also the size of molecules. Rate of migration increases with increase in number of charges and decrease in size of molecules.

### Technique (Fig. 26.1)

The apparatus consists of two troughs filled with barbitone buffer solution (pH 8.6) through which electric current is passed. Cut Whatman No. 3 filter paper into strips of 2 cm width. Soak it in buffer solution. Blot the excess buffer over a filter paper and suspend it over the glass rod fixed in the apparatus. The two ends of the strip should dip in the buffer solution in the inner compartments of the two troughs. The outer compartments of the 2 troughs contain electrode through which current is passed. A drop of serum is mixed with a drop of bromophenol blue dye. Using a 0.1 mL pipette, apply 0.05 mL of the mixed serum as a fine streak on the center of the paper supported by glass rod. Close the chamber with the lid and switch on the current adjusting it to 180–200 volts. The moving boundary of the migrating proteins, stained blue can be seen moving towards anode. At the end of 5 hours run, switch off the current, remove the strips holding the ends, place them in the hot air oven with temperature 110°C for half an hour. Then remove the strips from the oven and place them in the bromophenol blue staining solution overnight. Next morning, wash the stained strips in 2% acetic acid solution twice or thrice to remove the excess stain. Then they are kept in a fixative solution of 2% sodium acetate in 10% acetic acid for 6 minutes. Then, dry the papers in the hot air oven for 15 minutes. If necessary, blue color can be developed further by exposing to ammonia vapor and observe the various bands.

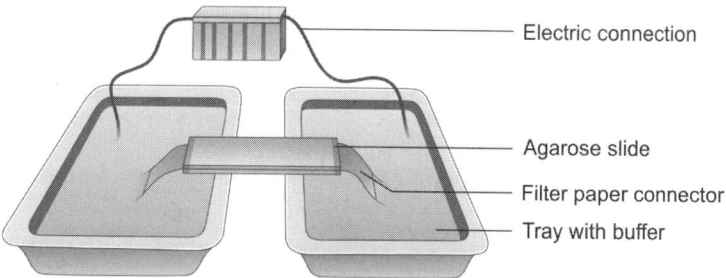

**Fig. 26.1:** Electrophoresis apparatus.

## Clinical Significance

Electrophoretogram of serum proteins is helpful in detecting changes in the individual protein fractions in serum and in detecting abnormal bands in certain diseased conditions. In a normal electrophoretogram the proportions of the various protein bands are as follows **(Fig. 26.2)**:
- Albumin: About 60%
- $\alpha_1$ globulin: About 4%
- $\alpha_2$ globulin: About 8%
- $\beta$ globulin: About 12%, and
- $\gamma$ globulin: About 16%.

The pattern in certain diseases **(Fig. 26.3)**:
1. Nephrotic syndrome
   Albumin          Reduced
   $\alpha_2$ globulin   Markedly increased
2. Chronic liver disease (cirrhosis liver)
   Albumin          Reduced
   $\gamma$ globulin   Increased.
3. Multiple myeloma: Abnormal paraprotein band in the $\gamma$ and $\beta$ region.
4. Agammaglobulinemia (congenital disorder)
   $\gamma$ band faint, Other bands – unaltered.

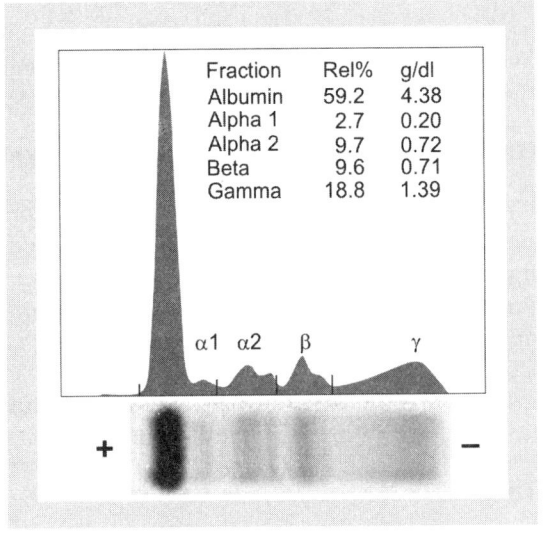

**Fig. 26.2:** Normal serum electrophoretogram.

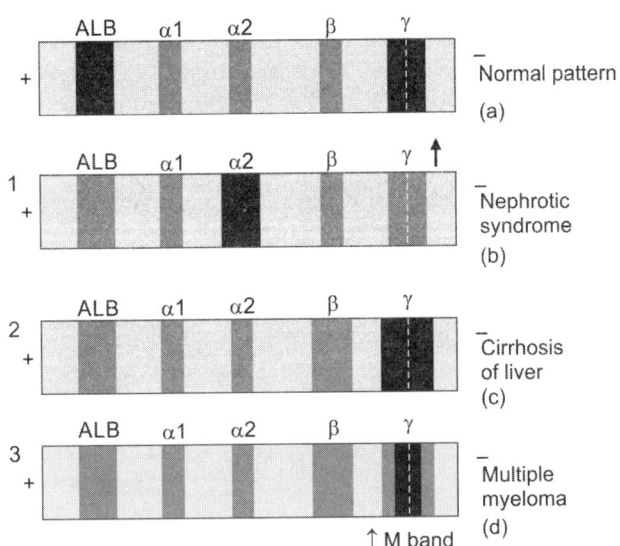

**Fig. 26.3:** Patterns of EPP in certain diseases.

# CHAPTER 27

# Polyacrylamide Gel Electrophoresis

| BI11.16 | Observe use of commonly used equipment/techniques in biochemistry including:<br>• pH meter<br>• Paper chromatography of amino acid<br>• Protein electrophoresis<br>• TLC, **PAGE**<br>• Electrolyte analysis by ISE<br>• Autoanalyzer<br>• DNA isolation from blood/tissue. |
|---|---|
| BI11.19 | Outline the basic principles involved in the functioning of instruments commonly used in biochemistry laboratory and their applications. |

## ■ POLYACRYLAMIDE GEL ELECTROPHORESIS (PAGE)

Supporting media for electrophoresis may be—Filter paper, cellulose acetate membrane, agar or agarose gel and polyacrylamide gel

- SDS: Sodium dodecyl sulfate -Polyacrylamide gel electrophoresis
- Polyacrylamide is produced by the polymerization reaction between acrylamide and methylene–bis-acrylamide (BIS) as catalyst.
- In PAGE electrophoresis, the anionic detergent—SDS is used to bind to proteins and give them electric charge.
- PAGE has high molecular sieving effect and so separation is very efficient.
- PAGE is widely used to separate biological macromolecules such as proteins and nucleic acids.
- Macromolecules will run in their native state or in denatured forms.

## Procedure

- **Preparation of sample:** Protein samples are heated with SDS detergent and mercaptoethanol to get a high negative charge.
- **Preparation of gel:** Polymerization of the gel is done by adding ammonium persulfate. BIS is added to form cross-links between acrylamide molecules in the gel. The mixture is degassed to prevent bubble formation.
- **Electrophoresis:** An electric current is applied to migrate the negatively charged proteins to the positive electrode. The migration depends on its molecular weight—smaller molecules

move more rapidly than the larger ones. At higher voltages, the migration is faster. Protein molecules will be separated by size within few hours.
- **Staining and visualization:** Staining is done by Coomassie Brilliant blue or ethidium bromide. Separated proteins will then appear as distinct colored bands.
- Unbound dye is then washed and dried.
- **Autoradiography detects the bands:** The proteins can be quantified—protein content is directly proportional to the quantity of bound dye.

## Applications

- To identify proteins
- To get purity of the sample
- To find the size of proteins
- To quantify proteins
- To identify disulfide bonds.

## Advantages

- Superior resolution
- Stable over a wide range of pH, temperature and ionic strength
- Simple speedy separation
- Electrically neutral and chemically inert
- Transparent to light
- Different pore-size gels can be made.

# CHAPTER 28

# Electrolyte Analysis

| BI11.16 | Observe use of commonly used equipment/techniques in biochemistry including:<br>• pH meter<br>• Paper chromatography of amino acid<br>• Protein electrophoresis<br>• TLC, PAGE<br>• **Electrolyte analysis by ISE**<br>• Autoanalyzer<br>• DNA isolation from blood/tissue. |
|---|---|
| BI11.19 | Outline the basic principles involved in the functioning of instruments commonly used in biochemistry laboratory and their applications. |

## ■ ESTIMATION OF ELECTROLYTES—BY FLAME PHOTOMETER

This is an analytical instrument used for quantitative analysis of sodium, potassium, calcium and lithium in biological fluids like blood, serum, urine, etc.

## Principle

The solution containing the substance to be measured is passed as a very fine spray into the air supply of a burner. In the flame, the solution evaporates and the substance is converted to the atomic state. As the temperature rises, the thermal energy of the flame excites these electrons so that they are able to absorb one more quantum of thermal energy and move into higher energy orbit further from the nucleus. The electrons in the higher energy orbits are prone to return to lower energy orbits. In doing so, the energy previously absorbed is released as quanta of light, the wavelength of which are characteristic of the substance thus giving rise to emission spectrum. Part of the light which is emitted in all directions is collected by a reflector and falls on a detector. The light intensity and hence the detector output is directly proportional to the concentration of the substance in the flame.

## Parts of the Apparatus (Fig. 28.1)

1. **Nebulizer:** It produces a fine spray of droplets of uniform size necessary for constant emission of light.
2. **Burner and flame:** When supplied with fuel and air at constant pressure (produced with the help of a compressor) the burner will produce a steady flame. If the sample is distilled water, the flame will be blue in color.

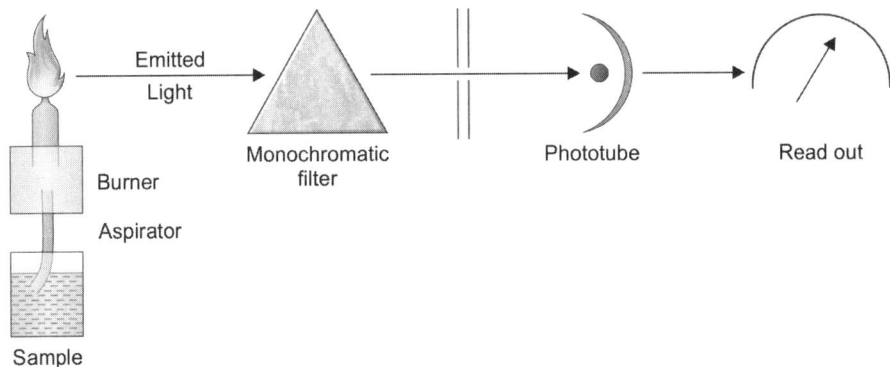

**Fig. 28.1:** Components of flame photometer.

3. **Capillary tube:** The free lower end is used to insert into the sample and the other end is focused over the flame.
4. **Filter:** Monochromatic filter. The principal wavelengths used are—589 nm for Sodium, 766 nm for Potassium—554 nm for Calcium, 671 nm for Lithium.
5. **Detector:** It is a photocell which converts light energy to electrical energy.
6. **Output devices:** Digital display or an external recorder. The amplified signal from the photomultiplier operates this device.
7. **Output tube:** To release the waste solution.

## Estimation of Sodium and Potassium in Serum by Using Flame Photometer: Preparation of Standard Solution

Stock solution: Sodium chloride: 0.85 g/L
Potassium chloride: 0.746 g/L

### Procedure

0.1 mL of sample serum is diluted to 10 mL with distilled water. Double distilled water is kept at the sample inlet. Standard and the test sample are also diluted as 1 in 10 dilution.

After switching the machine on, the air compressor is turned. The gas is opened and ignited. The apparatus is set to zero by using double distilled water. Then standard solution is kept and the reading is adjusted to 150 for sodium and 5 for potassium. Then the sample is fed and the readings are noted for sodium and potassium.

When the serum is introduced, the flame becomes yellow in color and the emitted light is focused onto the photocell after passing through the filters for desired elements. Reading is directly proportional to the concentration of ions.

## ■ ELECTROLYTE ANALYSIS BY ION-SELECTIVE ELECTRODE (ISE)

- This is an analytical instrument used nowadays for quantitative analysis of sodium, potassium, chloride, calcium, magnesium, bicarbonate and lactate in biological fluids like blood, serum, urine, etc.
- This instrument is relatively simple when compared to flame photometry which is having tedious procedures with high susceptibility to background interferences.

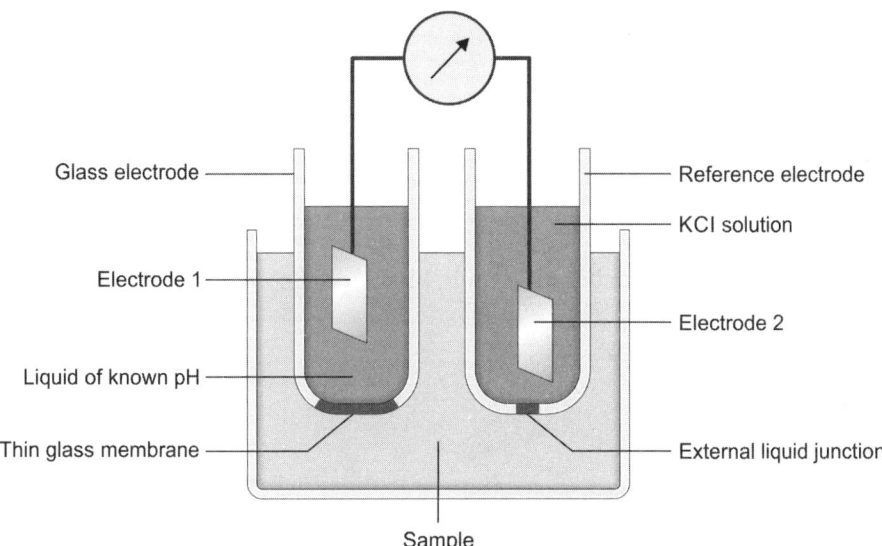

**Fig. 28.2:** Ion-selective electrode.

- This instrument is used in electrolyte analysis to assess:
  - The maintenance of acid-base balance
  - The maintenance of osmolality
  - The maintenance of fluid volume in different compartments
  - The muscle contraction and nerve impulse transmission.

## Ion-Selective Electrodes (ISE) (Fig. 28.2)

- In this instrument glass electrodes made of thin glass membrane are used which allow ions to permeate through. The electric potential difference (EMF – electromotive force) across the membrane is quantified by the machine.
- There are different electrodes used—each specific for different ions.
- Each electrode has a specific ion-selective membrane which undergoes specific reaction with the corresponding ions present in the sample to be analyzed.
- Different types of electrodes are membrane electrodes, liquid electrodes and solid state electrodes. The solid state electrodes are commonly used nowadays.
- The types of ion-selective membrane used commonly are glass, crystalline and ion-exchange resin membrane.

## Procedure

- A clear sample which is not hemolyzed should be used.
- The required amount of sample is sucked by the inlet capillary tube.
- Within few minutes the results are displayed and printed.
- Two readymade standards are used by the instrument—one high and one low standards with fixed concentration of analyte.
- The manufacturer's operation manual should be referred for proper procedure and result then and there.

## Interpretation

### Biological Reference Level

| Electrolytes | Serum (mEq/L) | Urine (mEq/L) |
|---|---|---|
| Sodium | 136–145 | 40–220 |
| Potassium | 3.5–5.0 | 25–125 |
| Chloride | 96–106 | 25–40 |

- **Hyponatremia:** Decreased sodium level in blood is called hyponatremia (Less than 130 mEq/L).
  **Causes:**
  - Vomiting, Diarrhea
  - Burns
  - Addison's disease
  - Renal tubular acidosis
  - Chronic renal failure
  - Congestive cardiac failure
  - Hypothyroidism
  - SIADH: Syndrome of inappropriate anti-diuretic hormone
  - Drugs: ACE inhibitors, Lithium, NSAIDs, Vasopressin and oxytocin
  - Pseudo or dilutional hyponatremia—Hyperproteinemia (Myeloma)
  
  **Signs and symptoms:** Dehydration, abdominal cramps, oliguria, tremors, and coma. May be asymptomatic.

- **Hypernatremia:** Increased sodium in blood is known as hypernatremia—more than 145 mEq/L.
  **Causes:**
  - Cushing's disease
  - Prolonged cortisone therapy
  - Dehydration
  - Exchange transfusion with stored blood
  - Primary hyperaldosteronism
  - Drugs—Anabolic steroids, oral contraceptives, diuretics.
  
  **Signs and symptoms:** Dry mucous membrane, fever, thirst, restlessness.

- **Potassium:** Potassium is the major intracellular cation and maintains intracellular osmotic pressure. Normal potassium level is 3.5 – 5.2 mEq/L.

- **Hypokalemia:** Plasma potassium level below 3.5 mEq/L is hypokalemia.
  **Causes:**
  1. Increased renal excretion: Cushing's syndrome, hyperaldosteronism, hyper-reninism, hypomagnesemia, renal tubular acidosis.
  2. Shift/Redistribution of potassium—alkalosis, insulin therapy, thyrotoxic periodic paralysis, hypokalemic periodic paralysis.
  3. Gastrointestinal loss—diarrhea, vomiting, aspiration, deficient intake, malabsorption
  4. Intravenous saline infusion in excess.
  5. Drugs: Insulin, salbutamide, osmotic diuretics, thiazides.
  
  **Signs and symptoms:** Muscular weakness, fatigue, muscle cramps, hypotension, decreased reflexes, palpitation, cardiac arrhythmias, and cardiac arrest. ECG waves are flattened, T wave is inverted. This may be corrected by oral feeding of orange juice.

**Treatment:** Adequate supplementation of potassium. About 100 mmol KCl per day in 3-4 divided dose.

- **Hyperkalemia:** Plasma potassium level above 5.5 mmol/L is known as hyperkalemia. Hyperkalemia is life-threatening. It is characterized by flaccid paralysis, bradycardia, and cardiac arrest. ECG—Elevated T-wave, widening of QRS complex, lengthening of PR interval.
  **Causes:**
  1. Decreased renal excretion of potassium: Urinary tract obstruction, renal failure, deficient aldosterone, heart failure.
  2. Entry of potassium to extracellular space: Increased hemolysis, tissue necrosis, burns, tumor lysis, crush injury.
  3. Redistribution of potassium to extracellular space: Metabolic acidosis, diabetes mellitus, tissue hypoxia.
  4. Hyperkalemic periodic paralysis.
  5. Drugs: Spironolactone, ACE inhibitors, beta blockers, cyclosporine, digoxin.
- **Pseudohyperkalemia:** Factitious, improper blood collection, thrombocytosis, leukocytosis.
  **Treatment:** When potassium level >6.5 mmol/L, intravenous glucose and insulin should be given. Continuous ECG monitoring should be done.
- **Chloride:** Chloride concentration in plasma is 96–106 mEq/L
- **Hyperchloremia:** Increase in serum chloride concentration.
  **Causes:**
  - Dehydration
  - Cushing's syndrome
  - Severe diarrhea leads to loss of bicarbonate and compensatory retention of chloride
  - Renal tubular acidosis.
- **Hypochloremia:** Decrease in serum chloride concentration.
  **Causes:**
  - Excessive vomiting
  - Excessive sweating
  - Addison's disease.

# CHAPTER 29

# Arterial Blood Gas Analyzer

| | |
|---|---|
| BI11.16 | Observe use of commonly used equipments/techniques in biochemistry including:<br>• pH meter<br>• Paper chromatography of amino acid<br>• Protein electrophoresis<br>• TLC, PAGE<br>• Electrolyte analysis by ISE<br>• **ABG analyzer**<br>• Autoanalyzer<br>• DNA isolation from blood/tissue |
| BI11.19 | Outline the basic principles involved in the functioning of instruments commonly used in biochemistry laboratory and their applications. |

## ABG ANALYZER (ARTERIAL BLOOD GAS ANALYZER)

Most of the severe and acute illnesses are associated with altered acid-base state. Rapid identification of the acid-base disturbance and correction is very important in the management of these cases. To understand the acid base disturbances, one should assess the biochemical parameters like pH, $PCO_2$, $PO_2$, bicarbonate and serum electrolytes. These parameters of blood gases like pH, $PCO_2$, $PO_2$, and bicarbonate levels can be quickly estimated by an instrument called blood gas analyzer. These are highly automated instruments consisting of ion-sensitive electrodes and potentiometers and greatly help the clinician to identify the acid-base disease state, so that corrective measures can be taken suitably and swiftly.

## Sampling

A heparinized arterial blood sample is collected from an artery, to determine arterial blood gases. Arterial blood sampling should be performed preferably by qualified health workers trained for the purpose. The sample can be obtained through a catheter placed in an artery, or by using a needle and syringe to puncture an artery. These syringes are preheparinized and handled to minimize exposure to air. During the procedure, radial artery can be punctured (**Fig. 29.1**) without using a tourniquet and let the arterial pressure push the plunger and fill the syringe. This is to avoid mixing of air in the sample which will interfere with the estimation of ABG. The syringe should be capped quickly to prevent contact between the arterial blood sample and the air, and to prevent leaking during transport to the laboratory. Firm pressure should be applied firmly to the puncture site to prevent bleeding and hematoma formation. The sample for ABG testing should be quickly transported to the laboratory for analysis of various parameters. Some of the components of ABG are measured directly and some are derived by calculations. Most blood gas analyzers offer automatic sample mixing and easy sample aspiration and automatic QC for accuracy.

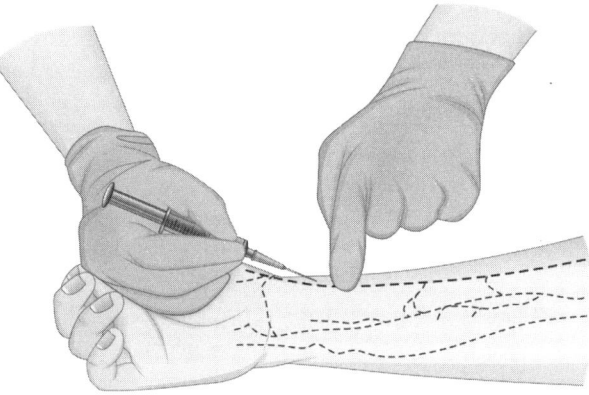

**Fig. 29.1:** Locate Radial artery and take a sample.

## Parameters Measured Directly

### pH

pH is measured with a glass electrode and a reference electrode suspended in the blood sample. The blood sample acts as a conducting electrolyte. The potential difference across the electrode varies proportional to the pH difference and this can be measured.

### $pCO_2$

$pCO_2$ is measured by a modified glass electrode. This electrode is bathed in a solution containing sodium bicarbonate (weak bicarbonate buffer). The $CO_2$ from the blood sample diffuses across a semipermeable membrane into the bicarbonate solution. This reaction changes the pH in the electrode and corresponds to a change in potential difference which is measured. The $CO_2$ concentration is inferred from the change in pH.

### $pO_2$

$pO_2$ level in arterial blood is assessed by electrochemical measurement of diffusion of $O_2$ through a permeable membrane into an electrode. This Clark's electrode consists of a silver anode and a platinum cathode which are immersed in an electrolyte buffer solution consisting of KCl and phosphate buffer. The reduction of oxygen at the cathode leads to a flow of current between anode and cathode. This is measured and is equated to assess the level of $O_2$ in the blood sample tested.

## Electrolytes

Serum electrolytes including Sodium, Potassium, Calcium and Chloride are determined by ion selective electrode techniques.

## Diagnosis of Acid-Base Disturbances by ABG

Based on the parameters received from the blood analyzer, we can find out the possible acid-base disturbance that is present in the patient. Looking at the pH, $PCO_2$ and $HCO_3$ one can diagnose the condition. If the pH is lower than normal, it suggests acidosis; and if higher, it denotes alkalosis. When this is because of alteration in $HCO_3$, the reason is metabolic. If the change in pH is due to change in $PCO_2$, it denotes respiratory disorder. The diagnostic criteria is summed up in the table below.

| Blood pH | $HCO_3$ | $pCO_2$ | Conditions | Causes |
|---|---|---|---|---|
| Less than 7.4 | Low | Low | Metabolic acidosis | • Kidney failure<br>• Diabetic ketoacidosis |
| More than 7.4 | High | High | Metabolic alkalosis | • Prolonged vomiting<br>• Gastric aspiration |
| Less than 7.4 | High | High | Respiratory acidosis | • Lung diseases<br>• Stroke |
| More than 7.4 | Low | Low | Respiratory alkalosis | • Liver failure<br>• Hysterical causes |

Though these blood gas measurements are used as a means of quantifying the severity of the acid-base disorder, patient's clinical history and the findings are the most important factors in deciding the cause of the disorder and will help to plan the corrective treatment.

| Acid-base disorder | Primary response | Expected compensation |
|---|---|---|
| Metabolic acidosis | Fall of $HCO_3$ | Fall of $PCO_2$ |
| Metabolic alkalosis | Rise of $HCO_3$ | Rise of $PCO_2$ |
| Respiratory acidosis | Rise of $PCO_2$ | Rise of $HCO_3$ |
| Respiratory alkalosis | Fall of $PCO_2$ | Fall of $HCO_3$ |

**Detection of compensation:** Primary metabolic disturbances elicit compensatory respiratory responses to maintain normal pH. In an acid-base disturbance, the compensatory response is in the same direction. For example, decreased $HCO_3$ leads to decreased $PCO_2$ and this is known as the **same direction rule (see Table above).** One should remember the range of compensation which will help to identify simple from mixed acid-base disturbances.

# CHAPTER 30

# Enzyme-Linked Immunosorbent Assay

| BI11.16 | Observe use of commonly used equipment/techniques in biochemistry including:<br>• pH meter<br>• Paper chromatography of amino acid<br>• Protein electrophoresis<br>• TLC, PAGE<br>• Electrolyte analysis by ISE<br>• Autoanalyzer<br>• **ELISA**<br>• DNA isolation from blood/tissue. |
|---|---|
| BI11.19 | Outline the basic principles involved in the functioning of instruments commonly used in biochemistry laboratory and their applications. |

## ■ ENZYME-LINKED IMMUNOSORBENT ASSAY (ELISA)

It is a non-isotope immunoassay. ELISA is used widely to measure hormone, growth factors, tumor markers, bacterial and viral antigens, etc. Here the antigen is labeled with a stable enzyme whereas in radioimmunoassay a radioisotope is used.

## Principle

- Enzymes used as labels catalyze color change in the substrate which is then detected.
- The amount of enzyme-labeled antigen bound is inversely proportional to the amount of antigen in the serum being analyzed.
- Commonly used enzyme substrate combinations are: Alkaline phosphatase with substrate p-nitrophenyl and Horseradish peroxidase with tetramethylbenzidine
- Two types of ELISA
  - Antibody detection—indirect ELISA (Single antibody)
  - Antigen detection—sandwich ELISA (Double antibody).

  1. **Antibody detection: Indirect ELISA (Fig. 30.1A):**
     - This is used to detect small quantities of antibodies.
     - HIV antibody is detected by this method.
       1. Specific antigen to the antibody coated well is taken.
       2. Then the sample (serum) is added and incubated. The antibody in patient's sample binds to the antigen and fixed.

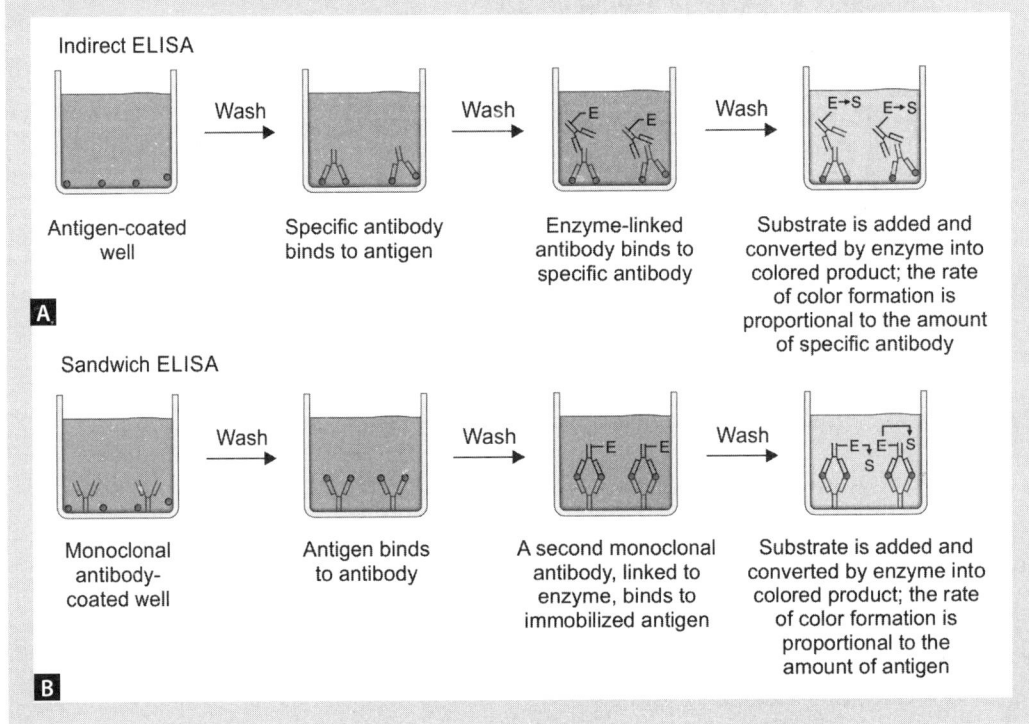

**Figs. 30.1A and B:** ELISA.

3. Next a second antibody conjugated with the enzyme peroxidase is added to the antigen-antibody already formed. Remaining is washed.
4. Now the Ag-Ab-Ab-Enz complex is obtained.
5. Now a substrate for the enzyme which will form a colored product is added. The color developed is directly proportional to the concentration of the analyte antibody.

2. **Antigen detection: Sandwich ELISA (Fig. 30.1B)**
   - Assay of thyroid hormone is done by this method.
     1. Specific antibody is fixed to the antigen coated well of a microtiter plate.
     2. Sample is added to the well and incubated at 37°C. The antigen in patient's sample is fixed to the antibody. Excess antigen is washed out.
     3. Next a specific antibody tagged with an enzyme like Horseradish peroxidase is added which will bind to the antigen (secondary Ag). Remaining is washed.
     4. The Ab-Ag-Ab-Enz complex is now obtained.
     5. Then a substrate for the enzyme which will form a colored product is added. The color developed is directly proportional to the concentration of the analyte antigen.
   - Radioimmunoassays (RIA): Instead of enzymes and color-forming substrates in ELISA, RIA uses radiolabeled substrates which emit radiation which is proportional to the concentration of the analyte (direct method).

# CHAPTER 31

# Immunodiffusion

| BI11.16 | Observe use of commonly used equipment/techniques in biochemistry including:<br>• pH meter<br>• Paper chromatography of amino acid<br>• Protein electrophoresis<br>• TLC, PAGE<br>• Electrolyte analysis by ISE<br>• Autoanalyzer<br>• **Immunodiffusion**<br>• DNA isolation from blood/tissue. |
|---|---|
| BI11.19 | Outline the basic principles involved in the functioning of instruments commonly used in biochemistry laboratory and their applications. |

## ■ PRINCIPLE OF IMMUNODIFFUSION

Immunodiffusion refers to the movement of the antigen or antibody or both antigen and antibody molecule in a diffusion support medium. It is a diagnostic laboratory test which detects the diffusion pattern through a substance such as agar or agarose gel.

The test is based on the principle of interactions between specific antigen (Ag) and antibody (Ab) leading to antigen-antibody complex formation. The formation of antigen-antibody complexes is used for qualitative and quantitative assessment of antigens and antibodies.

Two types of reactions of antigen and antibody leading to antigen-antibody complex formation are known. They are precipitation and agglutination.

When a soluble antigen reacts with an antibody it forms an antigen-antibody complex which can be seen as an insoluble precipitate. This reaction is called **precipitation** and is used to identify antibody or antigens using known counterparts. When a particulate antigen binds to a specific antibody under suitable conditions of pH, electrolytes and temperature, antigen-antibody complexes are formed visible to the naked eye as clump. This is called **agglutination.** These principles form the basis of **immuodiffusion** tests used in the laboratory to identify antigens and antibodies.

The commonly known techniques of immunodiffusion are:
1. Single diffusion in one dimension (Oudin procedure)
2. Double diffusion in one dimension (Oakley Fulthorpe procedure)
3. Single diffusion in two dimensions (Mancini procedure)
4. Double diffusion in two dimensions (Ouchterlony double diffusion)

- **Single immunodiffusion in one dimension (Oudin technique):**
  Here the antigen or antibody is fixed and the other one moves. Antibody is incorporated in agar gel and the antigen is added on top. This antigen diffuses down and a line of precipitation is formed.
- **Double immunodiffusion in one dimension (Oakley Fulthorpe technique):**
  Here the antibody is incorporated in the agar gel over which a plain agar gel layer is laid. When the antigen is layered over the agar gel, both the antigen and the antibody move towards each other resulting in a line of precipitation in the center of agar gel.
- **Single immunodiffusion in two dimensions (Mancini technique) (Fig. 31.1):**
  Here the antigen is placed in a well cut in the agar gel containing antibody. The antigen then diffuses out resulting in antigen antibody precipitate. The diameter of the ring is directly proportional to the concentration of antigen present.
- **Double immunodiffusion in two dimensions (Fig. 31.2):**
  Here both antigen and antibody are placed in the agar gel. A well cut in the center of the gel is filled with antibody. Two small wells are made on either side of this, and different antigens are added to these well. The movement of the antigen and antibody results in formation of antigen-antibody complex and forms a precipitation line. The pattern of lines decides whether the antigens are identical, partially identical or nonidentical.

## Clinical Uses

Immunodiffusion technique is used to identify antigen and antibody. It can be used to assess the concentration of antibodies in disorders of gamma globulin. Clinical use is in conditions like multiple myeloma.

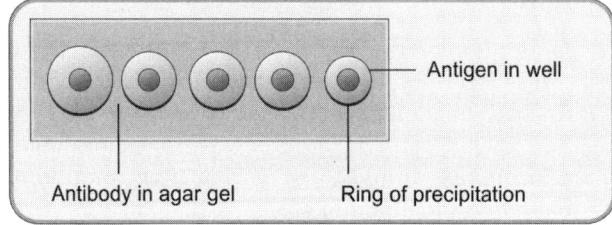

**Fig 31.1:** Single immunodiffusion in two dimensions.

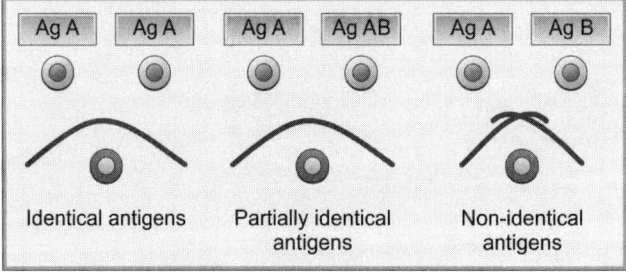

**Fig. 31.2:** Double immunodiffusion in two dimensions.

# CHAPTER 32

# Autoanalyzer

| BI11.16 | Observe use of commonly used equipment/techniques in biochemistry including:<br>• pH meter<br>• Paper chromatography of amino acid<br>• Protein electrophoresis<br>• TLC, PAGE<br>• Electrolyte analysis by ISE<br>• **Autoanalyser**<br>• DNA isolation from blood/tissue. |
|---|---|
| BI11.19 | Outline the basic principles involved in the functioning of instruments commonly used in biochemistry laboratory and their applications. |

## ■ AUTOMATED TECHNIQUES—AUTOANALYZERS

Awareness of monitoring good health has been increased nowadays and analysis of laboratory results help in arriving at the diagnosis and in monitoring of diseases at the shortest period. In major hospitals where large number of samples have to be analyzed every day, automation makes the work easier to get an accurate and quicker results.

Automation is based on the process by which many tests are done by lesser involvement of manpower with automatic control.

Autoanalyzers are automatic machines used in the biochemical laboratory to tackle the increased load under good condition **(Fig. 32.1)**.

## Semi-autoanalyzers

In this type, some steps are done manually such as pipetting of samples, mixing of reagents and incubation. The results are displayed and printed automatically. Only one analysis can be done at a time but many samples can be measured.

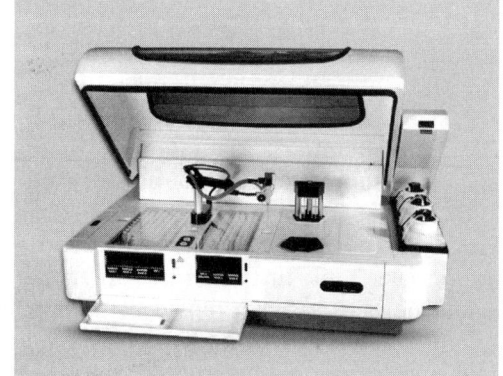

**Fig. 32.1:** Autoanalyzer.

## Fully Automated Analyzers

These may be of two types:
1. **Continuous flow:** Autoanalyzers in which the reagents and diluent are pumped through different tubings. Samples are sent along through the same pipeline and mixed with air bubbles. Output from these is displayed on a recorder – Not used nowadays.
2. **Discrete analyzers:** This may be either a) Discrete or b) Random access analyzer or Selective analyzer.
   a. *Batch analyzer:* Here, each sample is analysed for one particular test, e.g., Glucose or urea and the test is done for all samples.
   b. *Random access analyzer or selective analyzer:* It is the most sophisticated system which can analyse more number (40 or more) of parameters in a single sample—sample oriented. And also it is scheduled to analyze many samples at a time.

## Profiles of Analyzers

1. Accurate measurement and transfer of samples
2. Mixing with required volume of reagents
3. Incubation
4. Measurement of end point by absorbance
5. Calculation.

## Parts (Modules) of Autoanalyzer

A. **Sampler:** It has a base having a motor on which a circular tray with equally spaced holes is present. These holes can hold plastic cups to keep the samples. A probe connected by plastic tubing to the proportionating pump enters each sample serially. From the sample the probe passes into a wash reservoir.
B. **Proportioning pump:** (Similar to pipetting in manual method)
   It involves the peristaltic action done by a series of rollers on plastic pump tuber. Pumps will work at slow or fast speed. Air or fluid will be pushed forward when the roler passes along with the tubes. The volume of the samples/ reagent will be determined by the internal diameter of the tube.
C. **Dialyzer:** It is a semi-permeable membrane which separates big and small molecules when the stream of liquid passes through. Diffusible substances including the substance (analyte) passes through the membrane in the lower half into the recipient stream of reagents. The rest of the sample may go waste or it will be used for analyzing another constituent.
D. **Mixing chamber:** By vibration of probes, the reagents are mixed in cuvettes.
E. **Incubation bath:** It maintains the reaction of mixture at constant temperature—usually at 37°C or 90°C or higher.
F. **Flow through colorimeter and recorder:** Finally the stream of fluid passes through the opto-electronic instruments. Earlier the analyzers were used with colorimetric methods. But now it has been replaced by devices like spectrophotometers, fluorometers, flame photometers or radioactive counters. Results are prepared by the software attached after taking the absorbance.
Complete instructions and information about the instrument are supplied by the manufacturers.

## Advantages of Autoanalyzers

- Chances of manual errors are reduced and so results are accurate and reliable.
- The analyzers are based on computer and so they are self-monitored.
- Easy to operate.
- Workload can be finished in a short span of time.
- No need for manual calculations. Results can be digitally displayed and printed easily.
- Expenses per test are lesser when compared to other methods.
- All types of tests for all organ functions can be done at a time within a short period.

## Drawbacks of Autoanalyzers

- High cost of the equipment
- Errors in instrument
- Problems in power supply and in maintenance.

# CHAPTER 33

# DNA Isolation from Blood/Tissues

> **BI11.16** Observe use of commonly used equipment/techniques in biochemistry including:
> - pH meter
> - Paper chromatography of amino acid
> - Protein electrophoresis
> - TLC, PAGE
> - Electrolyte analysis by ISE
> - Autoanalyzer
> - **DNA isolation from blood/tissue.**

## ■ DNA ISOLATION FROM BLOOD/TISSUE

Pure DNA isolation from blood and tissues is highly essential for most of the genetic engineering technology to diagnose many diseases like inborn errors of metabolism, leukemias and also for prenatal diagnosis.

## Steps of Extraction of DNA

1. Lysis of cells after a short incubation period.
2. Purification and separation of DNA from other cell components.
3. Isolation of DNA by elution/precipitation with ethanol.
4. Quantification of DNA.

### *Precaution*

- Freshly collected whole blood is used.
- All steps should be carried out at room temperature.
- Centrifugation should be done in ultracentrifuge.
- Sterile micropipette tips should be used.

### *Procedure*

- **Step 1:** Lysis of red blood cells:
  - 20 μL of proteinase K is taken in a dry clean 1.5 mL centrifuge tube.
  - 200 μL of whole human blood in EDTA is added and mixed well.
  - 200 μL of lysis buffer is added and mixed well by vortex.

- **Step 2:** Separation of white blood cells:
  - 200 µL of 100% ethanol is added and mixed by vortex and then centrifuged to get a clear red supernatant and white blood cell pellet. The supernatant is removed.
- **Step 3:** Lysis of white blood cells:
  - To the WBC pellet, 200 µL of cell lysis buffer is added along with 50 µL of ammonium acetate and vortexed and centrifuged to get a protein pellet.
- **Step 4:** Separation of DNA:
  - The supernatant is transferred to another tube containing isopropanol.
  - This is mixed well many times till fine threads or clumps are visible.
  - This is again centrifuged and the supernatant is drained carefully to an absorbent paper to get the DNA pellet.
- **Step 5:** Extraction of DNA:
  - Wash buffers with ethanol are added to this DNA pellet and washed.
  - 100 µL of elution buffer is added and centrifuged at 8000 rpm for one minute.
  - The purity of the DNA is checked by using spectrophotometer at a wavelength of 260 nm.

## *Applications of DNA Isolation*

- Gene cloning
- To predict the virulence of microorganisms
- To identify the sources of hospital-based and community-based diseases.
- Identification of accused in rapes, accidents, paternity determination and war victims in forensic laboratories.

# SECTION 5

# Function Tests

## Section Outline

34. Gastric Function Tests and Analysis of Gastric Juice
35. Pancreatic Function Tests
36. Liver Function Tests
37. Analysis of Bile
38. Renal Function Tests
39. Thyroid Function Tests
40. Adrenal Function Tests

# CHAPTER 34

# Gastric Function Tests and Analysis of Gastric Juice

**PY4.8** Describe and discuss gastric function tests, pancreatic exocrine tests and liver function tests.

## GASTRIC FUNCTION TESTS

The functions of stomach include:
- Promoting digestion by its churning ability
- Reservoir of ingested food
- Stimulating the release of bile and pancreatic juice.

The gastric mucosa contains different types of cells to perform different functions:
i. Parietal or oxyntic cells—secrete HCl (pH 0.8)—by potassium activated ATPase enzyme. ATP is hydrolyzed to produce $H^+$ in exchange of $K^+$. The hydrogen ion is secreted into the gastric lumen which then combines with chloride ion which is produced in exchange of bicarbonate to secrete hydrochloric acid.
ii. Surface epithelial cells—secrete mucus.
iii. Chief cells or peptic cells—secrete enzymes like pepsin.

- The gastric juice is highly acidic in nature. It is clear, odorless, pale yellow, yellow fluid, having a pH of 1–2.
- Secretion of HCl is stimulated by a peptide hormone gastrin secreted by the G cells and by histamine which acts through $H_2$ receptors.
- HCl helps in activation of pepsinogen to pepsin and for absorption of iron and calcium.
- Gastric juice also contains a glycoprotein—the intrinsic factor which helps in absorption of vitamin $B_{12}$.
- Gastric juice contains 99% water and 1–2% solids. Solids include inorganic salts, mucin, and digestive enzymes like pepsin, renin and gastric lipase.
- The daily output varies from 2–4 liters. The abnormal constituents include lactic acid, blood, bile salt and bile pigment.
- Ryle's tube is used to aspirate the gastric contents.

## Assessment of Gastric Function

1. **Functional test meal (FTM):**
   - The collection of gastric juice is done by Ryle's tube aspiration under fasting condition and after taking a test meal in every 15 minutes for 2 hours. The samples are analyzed for free and total acidity. Free acidity denotes only hydrochloric acid; Total acidity represents the sum of free acidity and combined acidity of other organic acids like lactic acid, butyric acid and protein-bound $H^+$ ion, etc.
   Titration of gastric juice is done with N/10 sodium hydroxide, using Topfer's indicator for free acidity and phenolphthalein as indicator for total acidity.
   - FTM is not done nowadays, instead some modified procedures like pentagastrin stimulation test are being adopted.
2. **Pentagastrin stimulation test:**
   Pentagastrin is a synthetic peptide of 9 amino acids which can stimulate gastric secretion.
   - In fasting condition, stomach contents are aspirated by Ryle's tube – Residual juice.
   - For the next one hour gastric juice secreted is collected—known as basal secretion.
   - Stimulation of gastric secretion is done by giving pentagastrin 0.5 µg/kg body weight.
   - Gastric juice is collected at every 15 minutes interval for one hour—maximum secretion.
   - The samples are measured for basal acid and maximal acid output (BAO and MAO) by titration with N/10 NaOH using a drop of phenolphthalein as indicator.
   - Normal BAO: 1 – 2.5 mmol/h; MAO: 20 to 40 mmol/h.
3. **Augmented histamine test:**
   Basal gastric secretion is collected for one hour. 0.04 mg/kg body weight of histamine is given subcutaneously. Gastric secretions are aspirated then for next one hour at fifteen minutes interval. In all the samples the acid content is measured.
4. **Serum gastrin level:** Measured by ELISA
5. **Qualitative analysis of gastric juice**

| Experiment | Observation | Inference |
| --- | --- | --- |
| **A. Normal constituents (hydrochloric acid)** | | |
| **1. Topfer's test for hydrochloric acid** | | |
| 2 mL of gastric juice is taken in a test tube and 2 drops of Topfer's indicator is added and mixed. | Red color is seen. | Indicates the presence of hydrochloric acid. |
| **B. Abnormal constituents** | | |
| **1. Iodine test for starch** | | |
| To 2 mL of gastric juice, add few drops of iodine. | Blue color is formed. | Indicates the presence of starch due to the stasis of food in stomach as in duodenal ulcer or due to delayed emptying of stomach. |
| **2. Benzidine test for blood** | | |
| To a pinch of benzidine powder, 1 mL of glacial acetic acid is added and dissolved. Then 1 mL of hydrogen peroxide is added to it and then 1 mL of gastric juice is added. | Blue or green color develops which turns to brownish black in color within few minutes. | This shows the presence of blood in gastric juice which may be due to gastric ulcer or carcinoma of stomach or due to injury. |

*(Contd...)*

(Contd...)

| Experiment | Observation | Inference |
|---|---|---|
| **3. Test for bile** | | |
| **a. Hay's test for bile salts:** | | |
| Two test tubes are taken. In the first tube 2 mL of gastric juice and in the second 2 mL of water are taken. A pinch of sulfur powder is sprinkled over the surface of the liquid in each tube. | Sulfur powder sinks to the bottom of the tube containing gastric juice and floats in water. | Indicates the presence of bile salts in gastric juice. Bile could enter the stomach by regurgitation. Bile salts reduce the surface tension and hence the sulfur powder sinks. |
| **b. Fouchet's test for bile pigments** | | |
| To 5 mL of gastric juice few crystals of magnesium sulfate are added and dissolved by shaking. Then 2 mL of 10% barium chloride is added and mixed to get a precipitate. This is filtered in a filter paper and dried. Then 1–2 drops of Fouchet's reagent is added on the dry precipitate | A green color is developed. | Shows the presence of bile pigments. Bile enters the stomach by regurgitation. |
| **4. Test for lactic acid** | | |
| **a. Ufflemann's test** | | |
| To 2 mL of gastric juice, 2 mL of Ufflemann's reagent is added and mixed. (Ufflemann's reagent –1% Phenol + 10% $FeCl_3$) | Violet color is changed to yellow color. | Indicates the presence lactic acid. |
| **b. Maclean's test** | | |
| 2 mL of gastric juice is taken in a test tube and a few drops of Maclean's reagent (Containing mercuric chloride and ferric chloride) is added. A control is done with 2 mL of distilled water and few drops of Maclean's reagent. | Yellow color is developed in gastric juice. No color change in distilled water. | Indicates the presence of lactic acid which is formed due to the fermentation of carbohydrates because of the low HCl found in cancer of stomach. |

**Results:** The gastric juice contains..........................

## Interpretation

Increased gastric secretion:
- Zollinger-Ellison syndrome
- Gastric cell hyperplasia
- Chronic duodenal ulcer.

Decreased secretion:
- Gastritis
- Gastric carcinoma
- Pernicious anemia.

## Section 5: Function Tests

### Relevant Questions

1. What are the normal constituents of gastric juice?
2. Name the types of gastric cells and the various secretions secreted by them.
3. What is the pH of gastric juice?
4. Which cells secrete HCl?
5. What is the function of HCl?
6. Name the enzymes present in the gastric juice?
7. What is the daily output of gastric juice?
8. What is the function of pepsin?
9. What is the precursor form of pepsin?
10. What are the possible abnormal constituents of gastric juice?
11. In which diseases, blood will be present in gastric juice?
12. If lactic acid is present in gastric juice, what is it due to?
13. In which conditions bile will be present in gastric juice?
14. Which indicator is used to detect the presence of HCl in gastric juice?

# CHAPTER 35

# Pancreatic Function Tests

| PY4.8 | Describe and discuss gastric function tests, **pancreatic exocrine tests and liver function tests**. |
|---|---|
| BI11.17 | Explain the basis and rationale of biochemical tests done in the following conditions:<br>• Diabetes mellitus<br>• Dyslipidemia<br>• Myocardial infarction<br>• Renal failure, gout<br>• Proteinuria<br>• Nephrotic syndrome<br>• Edema<br>• **Jaundice**<br>• **Liver diseases, pancreatitis**<br>• Acid-base disorders<br>• Thyroid disorders |

## ■ PANCREATIC EXOCRINE FUNCTION TESTS

Pancreas is an endocrine as well as an exocrine gland. The endocrine hormones secreted by pancreas are insulin, glucagon and gastrin.

The exocrine pancreas secretes an alkaline fluid of pH 7 – 8.2 of volume around one to 2.5 liters under the control of the hormones secretin and cholecystokinin.

The major pancreatic enzymes are:
- Pancreatic amylase
- Pancreatic lipase
- Proteolytic enzymes – Trypsin, chymotrypsin, carboxypeptidase and elastase as their zymogens.

## Assessment of Pancreatic Function

A. Pancreatic enzymes assay:
   1. Pancreatic amylase:
     - Normal value: 50–120 units
     - This is estimated by Somogyi method manually.
     - In acute pancreatitis the level of amylase rises within 5 hours and reaches peak within 12 hours. The level returns to normal within 2–4 days. When the serum amylase level is falling, urinary amylase level started rising up.

- Clearance ratio (CR) = $\dfrac{\text{Urine amylase}}{\text{Sr. amylase}} \times \dfrac{\text{Sr. creatinine } (S_{cr})}{\text{U. creatinine } (U_{cr})} \times 100$

Normally the ratio is 1–4.4%. In acute pancreatitis the ratio varies from 7–15%

2. Lipase:
   - Lipolytic enzyme which hydrolyzes glycerol esters of long chain fatty acids.
   - Level is highly elevated in acute pancreatitis.

B. Indirect stimulation of pancreas:

Lundh test:
- Patient is asked to fast overnight. A duodenal tube is inserted through nose to reach the third portion of the duodenum and the tip is adjusted fluoroscopically. The content is drained into a cylinder kept in iced water 8 cm below the level of the patient. The resting juice is first drained and then a meal (containing 8 g of corn oil, 15 g casein and 40 g glucose in hot water to make total of 300 mL) should be taken within 15 minutes. The tube is drained for 2 hours and the volume is measured and hydrogen ion content is determined
- Normal hydrogen ion secretion is 12–20 mmol/min/mL
- In pancreatic insufficiency secretion is less than 10 mmol/min/mL.

C. Estimation of sweat electrolytes:
- It is a test for pancreatic cystic fibrosis in which sodium and chloride levels are increased in sweat.
- In this condition, there will be a thick viscous secretion of exocrine glands like pancreas, salivary, bronchial and sweat glands.
- Pilocarpine is injected into the skin to stimulate secretion of sweat glands. The sweat is absorbed by filter paper and the weight of the filter paper gives the weight of sweat. The volume of sweat is determined from the weight and specific gravity. The level of sodium and chloride are eluted and determined.
- Sweat chloride levels of more than 60 mmol/L on two occasions give the diagnosis of cystic fibrosis.

# CHAPTER 36

# Liver Function Tests

| | |
|---|---|
| PY4.8 | Describe and discuss gastric function tests, pancreatic exocrine tests and **liver function tests**. |
| BI11.17 | Explain the basis and rationale of biochemical tests done in the following conditions:<br>• Diabetes mellitus<br>• Dyslipidemia<br>• Myocardial infarction<br>• Renal failure, gout<br>• Proteinuria<br>• Nephrotic syndrome<br>• Edema<br>• **Jaundice**<br>• **Liver diseases, pancreatitis**<br>• Acid-base disorders<br>• Thyroid disorders. |

## ■ LIVER FUNCTION TESTS (LFTs)

- Liver is an important organ involved in metabolic and other biochemical functions.
- The tests used to diagnose liver diseases are called liver function tests. They are:
  1. Tests based on hepatic excretory function:
     a. Serum bilirubin—total and conjugated
     b. Urine bile pigments—bilirubin, bile salts, and urobilinogen
     c. Fecal urobilinogen
     d. Dye excretion test—bromosulfophthalein (BSP) test.
  2. Markers of liver injury—Estimation of liver enzymes:
     a. Serum alanine aminotransferase (ALT)
     b. Serum aspartate aminotransferase (AST)
     c. Serum alkaline phosphatase (ALP)—marker of cholestasis
     d. Serum gamma glutamyl transferase (GGT).
  3. Tests based on synthetic function: (Synthesis of plasma proteins):
     i. Estimation of proteins:
        a. Total plasma proteins
        b. Serum albumin, globulin, A/G ratio
        c. Prothrombin time.

ii. Estimation of lipids:
   a. Cholesterol
   b. Triacylglycerol
   c. Lipoprotein.
4. *Special tests:* (Metabolic liver diseases)
   Estimation of—
   a. Ceruloplasmin
   b. Ferritin
   c. Alpha-1 antitrypsin (AAT)
   d. Alpha fetoprotein (AFP).
5. Tests based on detoxification function: Estimation of—
   a. Blood ammonia and bilirubin
   b. Hippuric acid.

## Important Liver Function Tests

A. **Synthetic function:**
   1. Total plasma proteins, serum albumin, globulins:
      - Almost all plasma proteins with exception of immunoglobulins are synthesized by liver. Normal total serum proteins level is 6–8 g/dL.
      a. Albumin is quantitatively the most important protein synthesized by the liver, and reflects the extent of functioning liver cell mass.
         » Normal albumin level is 3.5–5.0 g/dL.
         » In hepatocellular diseases hypoalbuminemia occurs.
      b. Normal serum globulin level is 2–3.5 g/dL.
         » In chronic inflammatory disorders such as hepatitis and in cirrhosis of liver hyperglobulinemia will be present.
      c. A:G Ratio: Normal A:G ratio is 1,2:1 to 2.5:1
         » In all chronic diseases of liver, the albumin level is decreased. A reversal of A/G ratio is seen in cirrhosis of liver.
   2. Prothrombin time: (Synthetic function)
      - Since prothrombin is synthesized by the liver, it is a useful indicator of liver function.
      - The half-life of prothrombin is 6 hours only. Therefore PT indicates the recent function of liver.
      - PT is prolonged only when more than 80% of liver function is lost.
      - In Vitamin K deficiency, PT is prolonged.
      - To differentiate liver dysfunction from that Vitamin K deficiency, Vitamin K is given to the patient and PT is measured. Elevated PT even after administration of Vitamin K indicates liver dysfunction.

B. **Hepatic excretory function**
   Estimation of bilirubin: (Van den Bergh test):
   - The serum bilirubin estimation is based on van den Bergh reaction, where diazotized sulfanilic acid reacts with bilirubin to form a purple colored complex, azobilirubin. Normal serum does not give a positive van den Bergh test.
   - When bilirubin is conjugated, the purple color is produced immediately on mixing with the reagent, the response is said to be van den Bergh direct positive.

- When the bilirubin is unconjugated, the color appears only after addition of alcohol, so it is said to be van den Bergh indirect positive.
- When both conjugated and unconjugated bilirubins are present, it produces an immediate color, which intensifies on adding alcohol. It is then said to be biphasic.
- In hemolytic jaundice—unconjugated bilirubin elevated—so indirect positive.
- In obstructive jaundice-conjugated bilirubin elevated—so direct positive.
- In hepatic jaundice—both conjugated and unconjugated bilirubin elevated—so biphasic.

C. **Markers of liver injury – Estimation of Liver enzymes:**
  1. Serum alanine aminotransferase (ALT)/SGPT
     - Normal serum level of ALT: 13–35 U/L for males and 10–35 U/L for females
     - Its coenzyme is pyridoxal phosphate (PLP).
     - It is highly increased in toxic or viral hepatitis and moderately increased in cirrhosis and chronic hepatitis.
  2. Serum aspartate aminotransferase (AST)/SGOT
     - Normal serum level of AST: 8–20 U/L
     - Its coenzyme is pyridoxal phosphate (PLP)
     - It is a marker of liver injury and its level is increased in hepatitis and in cancer of liver. It is also a cardiac marker.
  3. Serum alkaline phosphatase (ALP): Marker of cholestasis
     - Normal level is 40–125 U/L.
     - Six isoenzymes of alkaline phosphatase (ALP).
     - Alpha-1 ALP, alpha-2 heat labile ALP, alpha-2 heat stable ALP, pre-beta ALP, gamma-ALP, leukocyte ALP (LAP).
     - They are due to the difference in the carbohydrate content.
     
     Increase in Alpha-1 ALP: Obstructive jaundice; alpha-2 ALP indicates hepatitis and pre-beta ALP indicates bone diseases, gamma-ALP—ulcerative colitis; LAP—increased in lymphomas.
  4. Serum gamma glutamyl transferase (GGT)
     - Normal level is 10–30 U/L.
     - It is increased in infective hepatitis and prostate cancers.
     - It is a marker of alcohol abuse. GGT is increased in alcoholics when other liver functions are within normal limits. It is decreased rapidly within few days of stopping alcohol. Increase in GGT is proportional to the amount of alcohol consumed.

# CHAPTER 37

# Analysis of Bile

> **BI11.17** Explain the basis and rationale of biochemical tests done in the following conditions:
> - Diabetes mellitus
> - Dyslipidemia
> - Myocardial infarction
> - Renal failure, gout
> - Proteinuria
> - Nephrotic syndrome
> - Edema
> - **Jaundice**
> - **Liver diseases, pancreatitis**
> - Acid-base disorders
> - Thyroid disorders.

## ■ ANALYSIS OF BILE

- It is the chief secretion of liver which is the largest gland in the body.
- It is stored in the gallbladder and discharged into the duodenum on demand.
- It is a golden yellow, viscous fluid.
- Daily volume of secretion is 500–1200 mL.
- pH of hepatic duct bile is 7.8–8.6 and gallbladder bile is 7–7.4. It is alkaline in nature.

## Composition

1. Water: 97%
2. Organic constituents: 2%
   a. Bile salts—0.7% (sodium and potassium salts of glyco/taurocholic acids)—derived from cholesterol
   b. Bile pigments—0.2% (Bilirubin)—Degraded product of heme
   c. Cholesterol—0.6%
   d. Lecithin—0.1%
   e. Fat and fatty acids—0.25%
   f. Glucose

g. Proteins—mucin, nucleoproteins
h. Enzymes—Alkaline phosphatase
3. Inorganic constituents—1%—Bicarbonates, chloride, sodium, and potassium ions.

## Factors Affecting Bile Secretion

a. **Choleretics:** Stimulate the secretion by liver, e.g. Bile salts, hormones—secretin, vagal stimulation.
b. **Cholagogues:** Stimulate the release of bile from gallbladder, e.g. cholecystokinin (This is stimulated by fatty acids, amino acids and calcium ions).

## Functions of Bile

1. Alkaline pH of bile neutralizes the acidity of the gastric juice.
2. Acts as surfactants and detergents for the digestion of fats to form micelles.
3. Excretes bilirubin which is the end product of heme metabolism.
4. Excretes cholesterol to regulate the body cholesterol pool.
5. Excretes drugs and metabolites after detoxification in liver.

## Analysis of Bile

| Experiment | Observation | Inference |
|---|---|---|
| **1. pH:** Test the pH with red litmus paper. | Litmus paper turns blue | pH of bile is alkaline |
| **2. Test for bile salts** <br> **a. Hay's test** <br> 2 test tubes are taken. In one test tube 3 mL of diluted bile is taken and in the other test tube 3 mL of water is taken as 'control'. Little quantity of sulfur powder is sprinkled over the surface of the liquid in each tube. Should not mix the contents. | Sulphur powder sinks to the bottom of the tube in bile and floats in water. | Indicates the presence of bile salts. Surface tension of bile is lowered by bile salts and so sulphur powder sinks. (This is useful in detecting bile salts in urine) |
| **b. Pettenkofer's test** <br> 3 mL of diluted bile is taken in a clean test tube and a little quantity of sucrose (table sugar) is added and dissolved. 3 mL of conc. sulphuric acid is added along the sides of the test tube. | A reddish purple ring is seen at the junction of 2 liquids. | Indicates the presence of bile salts. Sucrose is hydrolyzed and dehydrated by conc. $H_2SO_4$ to form furfural derivative which condenses with bile salt to form the reddish purple ring. |
| *Note:* This test is not used to detect bile salts in urine due to presence of interfering substances in urine. | | |

*(Contd...)*

(Contd...)

| Experiment | Observation | Inference |
|---|---|---|
| **3. Tests for bile pigments**<br>**a. Fouchet's test**<br>3 mL of diluted bile solution is taken in a test tube. Few crystals of magnesium sulphate is added and dissolved. Then 2 mL of 10% barium chloride is added and mixed. A white precipitate is formed which is then filtered by a filter paper kept in a funnel. The filter paper is then unfolded and dried by means of blotting by another filter paper. 1-2 drops of Fouchet's reagent is added on the dry precipitate. | Green color develops in the precipitate. | Shows the presence of bile pigments. The precipitate formed is barium sulphate which absorbs bile pigments. Ferric chloride present in the Fouchet's reagent oxidizes the bile pigments to give green colored pigment biliverdin. |
| **b. Gmelin's test**<br>5 mL of conc. nitric acid is taken in a test tube. Bile is taken in a 10 mL pipette and the pipette is inserted into the tube containing nitric acid and then bile is added to the nitric acid drop by drop. | Green, blue and brown colored rings are obtained. | Shows the presence of bile pigments. Bilirubin is oxidized by nitric acid to biliverdin (green), bilicyanin (blue), and bilifuscin (brown). |
| **4. Test for proteins in bile**<br>To 3 mL of diluted bile, few drops of glacial acetic acid is added. Little more acetic acid is then added. | Greenish white precipitate is formed which is not soluble in excess of acetic acid. | Shows the presence of nucleoproteins in bile. Excess of acid makes the precipitate insoluble by bile salts. |

**Result:** The reactions of bile are thus studied.

## Relevant Questions

1. What is bile?
2. What are its constituents?
3. Name the bile salts.
4. How do you classify bile salts?
5. How are the bile salts synthesized?
6. What is surface tension?
7. What is the action of bile salts on surface tension?
8. What are the uses of bile salts?
9. Name the bile pigments.
10. How are they formed?
11. What is the role of bile pigments?
12. In which disease bile salts and bile pigments are excreted more in urine?
13. Name the tests to detect bile salts and bile pigments in urine.

# CHAPTER 38

# Renal Function Tests

| | |
|---|---|
| PY7.8 | Describe and discuss **renal function tests**. |
| BI11.17 | Explain the basis and rationale of biochemical tests done in the following conditions:<br>• Diabetes mellitus<br>• Dyslipidemia<br>• Myocardial infarction<br>• Renal failure, gout<br>• Proteinuria<br>• Nephrotic syndrome<br>• Edema<br>• Jaundice<br>• Liver diseases, pancreatitis<br>• Acid-base disorders<br>• Thyroid disorders. |

## ■ Renal Function Tests (Kidney Function Tests)

## 1. General Tests

**Urine analysis:** Physical, chemical and microscopic examination
a. **Physical examination:**
   - Volume (24 hours urinary output)—**Normal: 1.5–2 L/day**
   - Appearance—Color
   - pH—**N-6.0**
   - Specific gravity—**N-1.015–1.025**
   - Osmolality
   - Smell
b. **Chemical examination:** Qualitative analysis for abnormal constituents of urine—mainly glucose, protein and blood
c. **Microscopic examination of the centrifuged sediment of urine:** For RBC, WBC, pus cells, crystals—to rule out urinary stones and casts.

## 2. Glomerular Function Tests

- Glomerulus acts as a sieve in filtering blood but it retains cells and proteins thus forming a glomerular filtrate—normally 170–180 liters/day. Out of this only 1.5 liters of fluid is excreted as urine and the rest are reabsorbed through the tubules.

- **Glomerular filtration rate (GFR): Normal GFR is 120–125 mL/min.** This is reduced in renal failure.
- **Clearance tests:** Done to assess the glomerular filtration and renal blood flow.
  - Renal clearance of a substance is the volume of plasma from which the substance is completely cleared by the kidney in one minute.
  - **Clearance** = mg of substance excreted per min/mg of substance per mL of plasma; $C = U \times V/P$   C = Clearance of the substance; U = Concentration of the substance in urine; P = Concentration of the substance in plasma; V = Volume of urine passed per minute.
  - Clearance is expressed as milliliter of plasma per unit time.
  - **Clearance tests:** This test is done by using either endogenous markers such as urea or creatinine or exogenous markers like inulin, $^{51}Cr$- labelled EDTA, $^{99}Tec$- labelled EDTA, etc. Out of all creatinine clearance test is the best.
  - **Creatinine clearance test:** It is based on the rate of excretion of metabolically produced creatinine which is excreted through urine. Creatinine is freely filtered by the glomeruli but not reabsorbed by the tubules. A small amount of creatinine is secreted by the tubules.
  - 24 hours urine is collected and blood is also collected for estimation of creatinine. Urinary volume is measured (V) and the concentrations of creatinine in urine (U) and plasma (P) are estimated and by using the formula $C = U \times V/P$ the creatinine clearance is calculated.
  - Normal range for creatinine clearance is 90 to 129 mL/min.
  - Reduced creatinine clearance indicates chronic renal damage and reduced blood flow to glomeruli.
  - **Normal urea clearance:** 75 mL/min.
  - **Normal inulin clearance:** 125 mL/min.

## 3. Tubular Functions Tests

**Renal** tubules reabsorb or secrete certain substances, concentrate the urine and acidify the urine. So it is important for maintaining specific gravity and osmolality of urine.
- **Specific gravity of urine:** Simplest test. Specific gravity of urine depends on the concentration of the solutes. In early stages of renal failure SG may be low due to kidney's inability to excrete solutes.
- Urine **concentration test (fluid deprivation test):**
  - Fluid intake is restricted for 15 hours. The first urine sample in the morning is collected and SG and osmolality measured.
  - If the SG is more than 1.025 or the osmolality exceeds 850 mosmol/kg, the renal concentration capacity is said to be normal.
  - Renal concentration ability is impaired due to tubular defect or in diabetes insipidus where there is decreased secretion of antidiuretic hormone.
- **Measurement of osmolality:**
  Measurement of urine and plasma osmolality is done by using osmometer. **Normal urinary osmolality ranges from 60 to 1200 mOsm/kg. Normal plasma osmolality is 285–300 mosm/kg.** The ratio between urine/plasma osmolality is calculated. Normal ratio is around 3–4.5. Urinary osmolality is decreased in diabetes insipidus.
- **Dilution tests:** This is done to check whether kidneys can excrete an excess water load. After emptying the bladder 1000–1200 mL of water is given to the patient. Hourly urine is collected

for next 4 hours. In each sample volume, specific gravity and osmolality are measured. A normal person will excrete all the water load within 4 hours. It is a more sensitive test.
- **Urinary acidification test:**
  (Acid load test – Ammonium chloride loading test)
  - This is used to diagnose renal tubular acidosis.
  - Ammonium chloride is given orally in gelatin capsule (100 mg/kg body weight) to induce metabolic acidosis. HCl produced is excreted as acidified urine.
  - Hourly urine collected for 2–8 hours and pH and acid excretion of each sample noted.
  - At least one sample should have pH lesser than 5.5. pH is not decreased in cases of renal tubular acidosis.
- **Fractional excretion of bicarbonate, sodium and phosphate in urine:**
  - Help in assessing renal tubular functions.

## Renal Threshold and Tubular Maximum

- Compounds whose excretion in urine is dependent on blood level are known as threshold substances.
- They are not excreted in urine when they are normal or low in plasma.
- When the blood level of the substance is elevated, the tubular reabsorptive capacity is saturated and the excess will be excreted in urine.
- The renal threshold of a substance is the plasma level above which the compound is excreted in urine. Renal threshold value of glucose is 180 mg/dL.
- The maximum reabsorptive capacity of the substance is known as the tubular maximum or Tm.

## Proteinuria

- Glomerular sieve will not permit bigger molecules having molecular weight more than 67000 D. But in glomerular damage which occurs in diseases like diabetic nephropathy the higher molecular weight proteins are also filtered and appeared in urine.
- Albumin is one of the first proteins to appear in urine due to glomerular damage.
- Types of proteinuria are glomerular proteinuria, microalbuminuria, overflow proteinuria, tubular proteinuria, etc.

### 1. Glomerular Proteinuria

Increase in filtered load due to glomerular damage and vascular permeability is called glomerular proteinuria.

### 2. Microalbuminuria

- It is also called minimal albuminuria or paucialbuminuria.
- When very minimal quantity of albumin (30–300 mg/day) is seen in urine it is known as microalbuminuria. This is an early indication of diabetic nephropathy and hypertensive nephropathy.
- Early morning midstream sample is preferred.
- It is expressed as albumin – creatinine ratio. Normal ratio in males is <23 mg/g of creatinine and in females -<32 mg/g of creatinine.
- It is measured by radial immune-diffusion or by ELISA.

# CHAPTER 39

# Thyroid Function Tests

| | |
|---|---|
| **PY8.4** | Describe function tests: **Thyroid gland**, adrenal cortex, adrenal medulla and pancreas. |
| **BI11.17** | Explain the basis and rationale of biochemical tests done in the following conditions:<br>• Diabetes mellitus<br>• Dyslipidemia<br>• Myocardial infarction<br>• Renal failure, gout<br>• Proteinuria<br>• Nephrotic syndrome<br>• Edema<br>• Jaundice<br>• Liver diseases, pancreatitis<br>• Acid-base disorders<br>• **Thyroid disorders**. |

## ■ THYROID FUNCTION TESTS

### Thyroid Hormones

- The thyroid gland secretes the hormones:
  1. Triiodothyronine: $T_3$
  2. Tetraiodothyronine: $T_4$ or Thyroxine
     They are produced by the iodination of the amino acid—Tyrosine present in thyroglobulin (TG) protein and stored there.
  3. Calcitonin (secreted by parafollicular 'C' cells): It decreases blood calcium level.

### Normal Values of Thyroid Hormones in Blood

- Free triiodothyronine: Free $T_3$: 80–220 µg/dL
- Free tetraiodothyronine: Free $T_4$: 0.8–2.4 µg/dL
- Total thyroxine ($T_4$): 5–12 µg/dL
- PBI: Protein bound iodine; Normal total PBI – 10 µg/dL
- It is the transport form of thyroid hormones in plasma and it is biologically inactive.

## Stimulation of Thyroid Secretion

- **Thyroid-stimulating hormone (TSH)** secreted by anterior pituitary gland. TSH – Normal level: 10 µU/L.
- It is increased in primary hypothyroidism; Decreased in primary hyperthyroidism.
- Thyrotropin-releasing hormone (TRH) of hypothalamus—stimulates the secretion TSH.

## Thyroid Antibodies

- They are thyroid-stimulating immunoglobulins (TSIg)
- Also called as long-acting thyroid stimulators (LATS)
- It is an antibody generated against TSH receptors.

## Metabolic Effects of Thyroid Hormones

- $T_3$ is more active than $T_4$.
- **Metabolic rate:** BMR is increased by increasing the cellular metabolism.
- **Thermogenesis:** Major effect—mediated through uncoupling of oxidative phosphorylation.
- **Synthesis of RNA and protein:** $T_4$ increases the synthesis of RNA and protein; $T_3$ causes protein catabolism and negative nitrogen balance.
- **Body weight:** Hyperthyroidism—Loss of body weight.
- **Glucose metabolism:** Increased gluconeogenesis and glycolysis.
- **Fatty acid metabolism:** Increased; Increased cholesterol and so level of cholesterol—decreased, which is an indicator of hyperthyroidism.

## Thyroid Function Tests (TFT)

A. **In Vitro TFT**
   - Total serum $T_3$ and $T_4$
   - Free serum $T_3$ and $T_4$
   - Blood TBG—Thyroid-binding globulins
   - Resin uptake test (T3RU)
   - Serum TSH
   - Thyroid autoantibodies
   - Serum cholesterol.
B. **In Vivo Tests:**
   - Thyroid iodine uptake
   - TRH and TSH stimulating tests.

## A. In Vitro Tests

### 1. Assay of Hormones

a. **Serum total $T_3$ and $T_4$ by immunoassay—RIA/ELISA**
   - $T_4$ levels are more reliable than $T_3$.
   - Normal $T_3$ = 70–200 ng/dL; $T_4$ = 5–12.5 µg/dL.
   - In hyperthyroidism, thyroid hormone levels—both $T_3$ and $T_4$ levels are increased but TSH levels decreased.
   - In hypothyroidism $T_3$ and $T_4$ are reduced in serum but TSH level is increased.

b. **Free $T_3$ and $T_4$—They are unbound thyroid hormones**.
   - More reliable test
   - Normal value of free $T_4$ = 10–27 pmol/L; $T_3$ = 3–9 pmol/L
   - ELISA techniques are used to quantitate this free fraction
   - Values increased in hyperthyroidism and thyrotoxicosis and decreased in hypothyroidism.
c. **Thyroid binding proteins—Thyroid-binding globulin (TBG)**
   - Normal level of TBG = 12–28 µg/mL
   - TBG—increased in hypothyroidism, pregnancy and in estrogen therapy; Level decreased in hyperthyroidism, nephrotic syndrome.
d. **Resin uptake test ($T_3$RU or $T_3$U)**
   - Indirect estimate of binding capacity of plasma TBG
   - Radioactive iodine labelled- $^{125}$I-$T_3$ is added to the patient's serum which will occupy the free-binding sites on TBG. Excess unattached $^{125}$I-$T_3$ is removed and the amount taken up by the resin is estimated.
   - Normal value of $T_3$U is 25–35%
   - Values increased in hyperthyroidism and decreased in hypothyroidism.
e. **Plasma TSH (RIA method)**
   - Most sensitive and reliable test of thyroid function tests
   - Level of TSH is inversely proportionate to $T_4$ and $T_3$ levels
   - Normal value = 2–6 µU/mL
   - In primary hypothyroidism TSH level is elevated due to lack of feedback but in secondary hypothyroidism, TSH and $T_3$ and $T_4$ levels are low.
f. **Thyroid antibodies**
   - To detect autoimmune disorders of thyroid gland caused due to the antibodies against thyroid tissues
   - Antibodies are produced against thyroid peroxidase and thyroglobulin in serum of patients having Hashimoto's thyroiditis and Graves' disease.

## B. In Vivo Tests

1. **Thyroid iodine uptake test**: Using $^{131}$I. Normal value – 1 to 13% absorbed after 2 hours and 15 to 45 and absorbed after 24 hours.
2. **TRH stimulation test:** TRH will stimulate TSH. If the hypothalamic–pituitary–thyroid axis is normal, the $T_3$ and $T_4$ secretion is increased. An abnormal response is observed in hyperthyroidism and hypopituitarism.
3. **TSH stimulation test:** IV administration of TSH will increase radioactive iodine thyroid uptake and blood thyroid hormone level.

### *Thyroid Scanning: Ultrasonography*

### Hyperthyroidism

- There will be increased rate of metabolism, loss of weight, tachycardia, fine tremors, sweating, diarrhea, emotional disturbances, anxiety and sensibility to heat.
- Causes of hyperthyroidism are toxic goiter, Graves' disease, excess intake of thyroid tablets, TSH secreting tumors of pituitary.
- $T_3$ and $T_4$ increased and plasma TSH decreased in all conditions. No response to TRH in Graves' disease and goiter and sluggish in other conditions.

## Goiter

- Enlargement of thyroid gland is called Goiter. There will be increased level of TSH. It is due to failure in autoregulation of $T_3$ and $T_4$ synthesis which may be due to excess of or deficiency of iodide.
- **Primary hyperthyroidism:** Seen in all the diseases of thyroid—Graves' disease, goiter, carcinoma, etc.
- **Secondary hyperthyroidism:** Due to diseases of pituitary or hypothalamus.

## Hypothyroidism

Two types of hypothyroidism—Primary and secondary
- **Primary:** Due to diseases of thyroid gland—autoimmune hypothyroidism, thyroidectomy and in congenital hypothyroidism
  - Lab. findings in primary hypothyroidism—Decreased level of $T_3$ and $T_4$ in blood, increased TSH in blood and exaggerated response to TRH.
- **Secondary:** Due to diseases of pituitary or hypothalamus—tumor or surgery
  - Lab. findings in secondary hypothyroidism—Decreased level of $T_3$ and $T_4$ in blood, decreased TSH in blood and no response to TRH.

## Myxedema

It is a condition of hypothyroidism in adults characterized by puffy face, lethargy and reduction in the mental and physical activities.

## Cretinism

It is a condition of hypothyroidism in children associated with mental and physical retardation.

# CHAPTER 40

# Adrenal Function Tests

| PY8.4 | **Describe function tests:** Thyroid gland, **adrenal cortex, adrenal medulla** and pancreas. |
|---|---|
| BI11.17 | Explain the basis and rationale of biochemical tests done in the following conditions:<br>• Diabetes mellitus<br>• Dyslipidemia<br>• Myocardial infarction<br>• Renal failure, gout<br>• Proteinuria<br>• Nephrotic syndrome<br>• Edema<br>• Jaundice<br>• Liver diseases, pancreatitis<br>• Acid-base disorders<br>• Thyroid disorders. |

## ■ ADRENAL FUNCTION TESTS

Adrenal glands are endocrine glands located above the kidneys one on each side. Each gland has got an outer cortex and inner medulla which are having different important biochemical functions of the body.

## Adrenal Cortex

The outer cortex is made up of 3 zones—each doing different functions
a. Outer most: Zona glomerulosa—production of mineralocorticoids—21C steroids promoting retention of $Na^+$ and excretion of $K^+$ and $H^+$ mainly in the kidneys.
b. Middle fasciculata.
c. Inner reticularis
   – Glucocorticoids and androgens.
   – Glucocorticoids are also 21C steroids—They are cortisol and corticosterone.
   – Cortisol is the predominant glucocorticoid hormone.
   – Androgen precursors.

## Functions of Glucocorticoids

- These hormones affect basal metabolism—mainly glucose and lipids and also promote protein and RNA metabolism.
- They are also involved in host defense mechanisms.
- Maintain blood pressure and stress response.

## Insufficiency of Glucocorticoids

1. **Primary insufficiency:** Addison's disease – This is characterized by hypoglycemia, low blood pressure, loss of appetite and loss of weight, impaired cardiac function. Plasma sodium levels are low and potassium levels are high with increased lymphocyte and eosinophil count. Increased pigmentation of skin and mucous membrane.
2. **Secondary adrenal insufficiency:** Due to deficiency of ACTH resulting from tumor, infarction or infections. Metabolic effects are the same as primary insufficiency but there is no hyperpigmentation.

## Glucocorticoids excess: Cushing's syndrome

This is due to prolonged use of steroids, tumors of adrenal cortex or pituitary.

This is characterized by hyperglycemia, muscle wasting, edema, osteoporosis and hypertension. There will be a peculiar distribution of fat with truncal obesity and buffalo hump. There will be delay in wound healing also. Added hypernatremia, hypokalemia and hypertension are due to mineralocorticoid action of cortisol.

## Primary aldosteronism (Conn's syndrome)

- This is due to small adenoma of the glomerulosa cells.
- The manifestations of this condition are hypertension, hypokalemia, hyponatremia and alkalosis.
- Plasma renin and angiotensin II levels are suppressed.

## Secondary aldosteronism

This resembles primary aldosteronism except for the elevated renin and angiotensin II levels. This is due to renal artery stenosis.

## Assessment of adrenocortical functions

1. Measuring of plasma cortisol level – Normal 5–15 µg/dL – by RIA/HPLC
2. 24 hours urine-free cortisol
3. Assay of plasma ACTH level
4. Dexamethasone suppression test
5. Assay of urinary 17-ketosteroids.

# Adrenal Medulla

Adrenal medulla and sympathetic ganglia produce catecholamines which include epinephrine (adrenaline), norepinephrine (noradrenaline) and dopamine. They are synthesized from the amino acid tyrosine.

## Actions of Catecholamines

- Epinephrine is released in response to flight, fight. Fright, exercise and hypoglycemia.
- Epinephrine and norepinephrine—increase blood pressure.
- Epinephrine increases the rate and force of cardiac contraction.
- Epinephrine causes relaxation of smooth muscles of bronchi.
- Epinephrine is anti-insulin in nature and it increases glycogenolysis and stimulates lipolysis.

## Degradation of Epinephrine

By methyltransferase and monoamine oxidase enzymes, epinephrine is degraded to 3-hydroxy-methoxymandelic acid or vanillyl mandelic acid (VMA) which is normally excreted in urine 2–6 mg/24 hours.

In pheochromocytoma or neuroblastoma the urinary excretion of VMA is increased.

Measuring catecholamines in blood and urine:
1. By HPLC methods
2. Fluorimetric determination
3. Urinary VMA estimation in 24 hours urine.

# SECTION 6

# Food and Energy

## Section Outline

41. Energy Content of Food and Glycemic Index
42. Fats in Food

# CHAPTER 41

# Energy Content of Food and Glycemic Index

**BI11.23** Calculate energy content of different food items, identify food items with high and low glycemic index and explain the importance of these in the diet.

## ENERGY CONTENT OF FOOD

### Caloric Requirement

- Energy expenditure can be determined directly by measuring heat output from the body but is normally estimated indirectly from the consumption of oxygen. There is an energy expenditure of 20 kJ/L of oxygen consumed regardless of whether the fuel being metabolized is carbohydrate, fat, or protein.
- **Calorific value** of nutrients (energy density) is measured by using Bomb Calorimeter. It is the energy yield per unit weight of food. More energy is produced from fat.
- **Respiratory quotient (RQ):** It is the measurement of the ratio of the volume of carbon dioxide produced in L/g to volume of oxygen consumed in L/g. Respiratory quotient is an indication of the mixture of metabolic fuels being oxidized. The calorific value of nutrients is shown in the table below.

|  | Energy (KJ/g) | $O_2$ consumed (L/g) | $CO_2$ produced (L/g) | RQ |
|---|---|---|---|---|
| Carbohydrate | 16 | 0.8 | 0.8 | 1 |
| Protein | 17 | 0.9 | 0.8 | 0.8 |
| Fat | 37 | 2 | 1.4 | 0.7 |

Energy requirement is calculated by:
1. Maintenance for BMR (basal metabolic rate)
2. Specific dynamic action (SDA)
3. Extra energy expenditure for physical activity.

1. **Basal metabolic rate (BMR):** The energy required by an awaken individual during physical, emotional and digestive rest. It is the minimum amount of energy required to perform vital functions such as circulation, respiration, working of heart, etc.
   **Normal value**
   Men: 34–37 kcal/m²/hr
   Women: 30–35 kcal/m²/hr

It is the energy expenditure by the body when at rest—but not asleep—under controlled conditions of thermal neutrality, measured at about 12 hours after the last meal, and depends on weight, age, and gender. It is therefore possible to calculate an individual's energy requirement from body weight, age, gender, and level of physical activity.

2. **Specific dynamic action (SDA)**
   - It is represented as thermogenic effect of food. The heat is produced after intake of food, which is due to energy expenditure for digestion, absorption and transport of digestive products. This is also called **Diet induced Thermogenesis**.
   - SDA can be considered as the activation of energy needed for various chemical reactions. This activation energy is to be supplied initially. This activation energy is varied to different food.
   - For example, for carbohydrate—5%, for proteins—30% and for fat—15%, etc.

3. **Physical activity**
   - Energy requirement of an individual depends upon—occupation, physical activity and life-style which can be divided into 3 groups—Sedentary, moderate and heavy.
   - Heavy workers need high BMR.

## Balanced Diet

It is defined as the diet which contains all the necessary food materials like carbohydrates, proteins, and lipids along with vitamins, minerals in adequate proportions to meet the body's need.

- The diet should be simple, locally available, palatable and digestible.
- Adequate protein content with essential amino acids should be supplied. This is achieved by cereals pulses mixture with additional animal proteins.
- Calorie intake should be correct and should balance energy expenditure (30–35 kcal/kg body weight).
- Special care should be taken to see that adequate quantity of calcium and iron are obtained from the diet.
- Should provide adequate roughage.
- Cereals and pulses ratio is maintained at 5:1.
- Daily requirement of protein is 60 g, fat—45 g, calories—2000 kcal, calcium—400 mg, iron—25 mg.
- Diet is divided into 3 meals per day, breakfast, lunch, supper.
- Balanced diet should contain calories from carbohydrates, protein and fat in the ratio 60:20:20.

## Energy Content of Foods—Calculation

This is calculated from the heat released by the total combustion of food in calorimeter. It is expressed in kilocalories (kcal/Cal) – Joules (J). 1 kcal = 4184 J.

Energy obtained from the primary nutrients:
- Carbohydrates: 4 kcal/g or 17 kJ
- Proteins: 4 kcal/g or 17 kJ
- Fats: 9 kcal/g or 38 kJ

## Glycemic Index of Food

- It is assessed by GTT (glycemic response) after a particular diet and compare it with a reference meal – 50 g of glucose
  Glycemic index =

$$\frac{\text{Incremental area under glucose tolerance curve after 50 g test meal}}{\text{Incremental area under glucose tolerance curve after 50 g of glucose (reference meal)}} \times 100$$

- Simple carbohydrates like glucose or sugar will have high glycemic index, e.g. White rice, cereals, potato-fries.
- Low GI foods: Oats, vegetables – lentils, carrot, etc.
- But the same amount of complex carbohydrates like starch or dietary fibers have lower glycemic index as the digestion and absorption of these carbohydrates are slow.
- Glycemic index of carbohydrates is lowered if it is combined with proteins, fat or fibers.

For example: Potato chips have high GI (85–90) whereas ice cream has lower GI (around 35) as it has lots of fats.

## Importance of Glycemic Index

Low glycemic index foods are preferred for the patients with diabetes mellitus—55% of carbohydrates, 25% of fat and 20% proteins. They should take more green leafy vegetables and avoid tubers. They should avoid sweets and refined carbohydrates. Frequent small meals are recommended for distribution of calories for diabetic patients.

# CHAPTER 42

# Fats in Food

**BI11.24** Enumerate advantages and /or disadvantages of use of unsaturated, saturated and trans fats in food.

## ■ SATURATED AND UNSATURATED FATS IN FOOD

Foods with lipids or fats contain more calories than that contain proteins and carbohydrates. More intake of lipids is a risk factor for atherosclerosis and diabetes mellitus.

The fat of our body is triacylglycerol (Triglyceride). It contains 3 molecules of fatty acid esterified to one molecule of glycerol and it is the storage form of lipid mainy in adipose tissues.

Lipids are classified as follows:
- Simple lipids
- Compound lipids
- Derived lipids.

**Simple lipids**: They are the esters of fatty acids with various alcohols.
They are esters of fatty acids with glycerol.

**Compound lipids:** Compound lipids are lipids + prosthetic group, e.g., Phospholipids

**Derived lipids:** Products obtained from hydrolysis of simple or compound lipids – Fatty acids, glycerol, etc.

## Fatty Acids

- **Saturated fatty acids** are linear chain fatty acids which do not have double bond in their hydrocarbon chain.
- **Unsaturated fatty acids** contain double bonds in their hydrocarbon chains. Depending upon the number of double bonds. They are subclassified into:
  - **Monounsaturated fatty acid, e.g.,** Oleic acid
  - **Polyenoic or Polyunsaturated fatty acid:** They are:
    - **Dienoic acid:** 2 double bonds, e.g., Linoleic acid
    - **Trienoic acid:** 3 double bonds, e.g., Linolenic acid
    - **Tetraenoic acid:** 4 double bonds, e.g., Arachidonic acid.

- Essential fatty acids cannot be synthesized by the body but have to be supplemented in diet. They are polyunsaturated fatty acids (PUFA) having more than one double bond. They are:
  1. Linoleic acid (18 C): ω6
  2. Linolenic acid (18 C): ω3
  3. Arachidonic acid (20 C): ω6.
- 'ω' or 'n' refers to number of carbon atoms from end methyl carbon.
- $\omega_3$ series represents the double bond position between 3rd and fourth carbon atoms. E.g. Alpha linolenic acid, eicosapentaenoic acid—found in fish oil, walnuts etc. They prevent heart diseases. They help in pregnancy and in brain function.
- $\omega_6$ series represents the double bond position between 6th and 7th carbon atoms. E.g. Linoleic acid, arachidonic acid. Sources are sunflower oil and soybean oil.
- $\omega_9$ series represents the double bond position between 9th and 10th carbon atoms. E.g. Oleic acid.

**Trans-fatty acids** are fats produced by hydrogenation, to stabilize polyunsaturated oils from rancidity. They contain double bonds in the trans configuration. They increase HDL cholesterol and decrease LDL cholesterol level. They are risk factors for atherosclerosis.

## Significance of PUFA

- They are present in vegetable oils and fish oils.
- Used for esterification and excretion of cholesterol.
- It increases the fluidity of membranes.
- Anti-atherogenic.

| PUFA | Carbon atom | Double bond | Family |
|---|---|---|---|
| Linoleic acid | 18 | 2 | Omega 3 |
| Linolenic acid | 18 | 3 | Omega 6 |
| Arachidonic acid | 20 | 4 | Omega 6 |

# SECTION 7

# Clinical Case Studies

## Section Outline

43. Basis and Rationale of Biochemical Tests Done in Certain Clinical Conditions

# CHAPTER 43

# Basis and Rationale of Biochemical Tests Done in Certain Clinical Conditions

> **BI11.17** Explain the basis and rationale of biochemical tests done in the following conditions:
> - Diabetes mellitus
> - Dyslipidemia
> - Myocardial infarction
> - Renal failure, gout
> - Proteinuria
> - Nephrotic syndrome
> - Edema
> - Jaundice
> - Liver diseases, pancreatitis
> - Acid-base disorders
> - Thyroid disorders.

## ■ BASIS OF BIOCHEMICAL TESTS DONE IN DISEASES

History of a case which can be diagnosed based on the biochemical laboratory findings will be given to the students. Relevant questions will be given related to the case and the students will be asked to write the answers. Possible patterns of questions:

A. What is the diagnosis of the case?
B. What are the points in favor of diagnosis?
C. What are the investigations which will give the clue to the diagnosis? Give their normal ranges.
D. What other biochemical investigations could be done for that case?
E. What is the probable cause for the disease?
F. How can that particular disease be treated? Prevented?
   - The student may be asked to do quantitative estimation of one of the relevant investigations suggested by the examiner.
   - Discussion of the case related to biochemistry will be done and the knowledge of the student regarding the case can be assessed. Some of the case histories are given below with probable questions.

## List of Clinically Important Cases

| S. No. | Types | Disorders | Subtypes |
|---|---|---|---|
| I. | Metabolic disorders | A. Diabetes mellitus | 1. Type 1<br>2. Type 2<br>3. DKA |
| | | B. Liver diseases—jaundice | 1. Neonatal<br>2. Hemolytic<br>3. Hepatic<br>4. Obstructive |
| | | C. Acid-base disorders | 1. Metabolic acidosis<br>2. Metabolic alkalosis<br>3. Respiratory acidosis<br>4. Respiratory alkalosis |
| | | D. Cardiac disease | Myocardial infarction |
| | | E. Renal diseases | 1. Nephrotic syndrome<br>2. Chronic renal failure |
| | | F. Purine metabolism | Gout |
| II. | Deficiency disorders | A. Vitamin A<br>B. Vitamin D<br>C. Vitamin C<br>D. Vitamin $B_{12}$<br>E. Protein-energy malnutrition | 1. Night blindness<br>2. Rickets<br>3. Scurvy<br>4. Megaloblastic anemia<br>5. Kwashiorkor |
| III. | Inherited disorders | A. Carbohydrate metabolism | 1. Lactose intolerance<br>2. Galactosemia<br>3. Hereditary fructose intolerance (HFI) |
| | | B. Lipid metabolism | Familial hypercholesterolemia (FH) |
| | | C. Amino acid metabolism | 1. Homocystinuria<br>2. Phenylketonuria (PKU)<br>3. Alkaptonuria |
| IV. | Hormonal disorders | A. Thyroid disorder<br>B. Parathyroid | 1. Hypothyroidism<br>2. Hyperparathyroidism |

# I. METABOLIC DISORDERS

## A. Diabetes Mellitus

### 1. Diabetes Mellitus—Type 1

**Case:** A thin and emaciated 14-year-old boy complains of passing urine frequently and not putting on weight in spite of taking good amount of food. His laboratory reports are given below:
- **Urine albumin** : Nil
- **Urine sugar** : +++
- **Urine ketone bodies** : Nil
- **Blood glucose (F)** : 210 mg/dL
- **Blood glucose (PP)** : 450 mg/dL
- **Blood urea** : 35 mg/dL

1. What is the probable diagnosis and what is it due to?
   Type 1 diabetes mellitus (IDDM).
   Due to decreased insulin production.
2. Which age-group is commonly affected?
   Young adults below 30 years of age.
3. What is type 2 DM?
   NIDDM—due to decreased response to insulin—insulin resistance.
   Commonly seen in adults above 40 years.

## 2. Diabetes Mellitus (Type II) NIDDM

**Case:** A 50 years old woman came to the medical OP with complaints of feeling weak and tired for the past 2 months. She also complained of feeling thirsty often and feeling hungry in between meals. She used to pass large quantity of urine often and even wakes up during night 2–3 times for micturition. She revealed that her mother and maternal uncle had diabetes mellitus.

Her biochemical reports are given below:
- Urine: Albumin: Nil, Sugar +++, Ketone bodies: Nil
- Blood: Glucose fasting: 180 mg/dL
- Glucose: Postprandial: 340 mg/dL
- Urea: 38 mg/dL
- Serum cholesterol: 280 mg/dL
- HbA1c: 14%

1. What is your diagnosis?
   Diabetes mellitus (Type 2) NIDDM (Non-insulin-dependent diabetes mellitus).
2. What is Type 2 DM due to?
   Due to decreased biological response to insulin—Insulin resistance.
3. Why is there polyuria?
   As the blood glucose level is higher than the renal threshold level (180 mg/dL) urinary glucose excretion occurs. To excrete this glucose load, increased urine volume is required. This is called solute diuresis.
4. What is HbA1c?
   It is glycated hemoglobin, which is a non-enzymatic addition of glucose to hemoglobin. Normally the level is less than 6%. It reveals the mean glucose level over the previous 10–12 weeks.

## 3. Diabetic Ketoacidosis (Metabolic Acidosis)

**Case:** A 60-year-old man was brought to the casualty in a comatose state. His breathing was rapid and deep and smelt of fruity odor. He was admitted immediately and his laboratory results were as given below:
- Urine: sugar ++++
- Urine ketone bodies ++
- Blood glucose: Random: 660 mg%
- Blood urea: 50 mg/dL
- Serum creatinine: 2 mg/dL
- Arterial blood gas analysis: pH 7.25; $pCO_2$: 32 mm Hg

- Serum Na⁺: 130 mEq/L
- Serum K⁺: 6 mEq/L

1. What is your diagnosis?
   Diabetes Ketoacidosis (Type II DM).
2. Why there is ketosis?
   Due to insulin deficiency, glucose is not entering the cells. So cells start metabolizing more fatty acids to meet the energy needs. More beta-oxidation leads to increased production of acetyl CoA which will be converted to high levels of ketone bodies.
3. Why is there hyperkalemia?
   Deficiency of insulin leads to hyperkalemia as insulin is needed for the uptake of potassium by cells. Ketoacidosis increases H+, K+ antiport causing increased efflux of potassium from cells.
4. What are the complications of DM?
   - Microangiopathy in small blood vessels
   - Atherosclerosis in medium-sized blood vessels
   - Cataract of lens in the eyes due to deposition of sorbitol
   - Retinal microvascular abnormalities lead to retinopathy
   - Nephropathy
   - Neuropathy.

## B. Liver Diseases: Jaundice

- Bilirubin is the end product of catabolism of heme. Normal value of total bilirubin is 0.2–0.8 mg/dL; unconjugated bilirubin is 0.2–0.6 mg/dL and conjugated bilirubin is 0–0.2 mg/dL.
- If the levels are increased, the person becomes jaundiced or icteric. There will be yellowish discoloration of sclera, conjunctiva, skin and mucous membrane.
- There are 3 types of jaundice – hemolytic (prehepatic) jaundice, hepatocellular (hepatic) jaundice and obstructive (post-hepatic) – due to acquired causes.
- Laboratory diagnosis of jaundice:

| No. | Tests | Hemolytic jaundice | Hepatic jaundice | Obstructive jaundice |
| --- | --- | --- | --- | --- |
| 1. | Serum total bilirubin | Increased | Increased | Increased |
| 2. | Sr. conjugated bilirubin | Normal | Increased | Increased |
|    | Unconjugated bilirubin | High | Increased | Normal |
| 3. | Van den Bergh | Indirect + | Biphasic | Direct + |
| 4. | Alkaline phosphatase | Normal | Increased | Highly increased |
| 5. | Urine – BS (Hay's test) | Nil | Nil | Present |
| 6. | Urine – Conj. bilirubin | Nil | Present | Present |
| 7. | Urine – Urobilinogen | Increased | Nil | Nil |
| 8. | Fecal stercobilinogen | Increased | Decreased | Absent |

1. Van den Bergh: Indirect: Unconjugated bilirubin in blood, positive for prehepatic and hepatic jaundice.
2. Direct van den Bergh test: Conjugated bilirubin in blood is positive—helps in detection of post-hepatic jaundice.

3. ALP: Normal range: 40–125 U/L—increases slightly in hepatic jaundice and more in post-hepatic jaundice.
4. Hay's test: This test is specific for identification of urine bile salts—positive for post-hepatic jaundice
5. Fouchet's test (conjugated bilirubin in urine): This test gives positive result for both hepatic and posthepatic.
6. Ehrlich test (for urobilinogens): Positive in prehepatic and positive in early stages of hepatic.

## 1. Neonatal/Physiological Jaundice

**Case:** A preterm male baby born 3 days ago developed jaundice which was increasing gradually and then after 2 days it subsided. The child was given phototherapy. The laboratory reports of the child are given below:

| Day | Total serum bilirubin | Conjugated bilirubin |
|---|---|---|
| 1st day | 3 mg% | 0.5 mg% |
| 3rd day | 8 mg% | 2.5 mg% |
| 5th day | 7 mg% | 3.5 mg% |
| 7th day | 2 mg% | 1 mg% |

1. What is the probable diagnosis?
   Physiological or neonatal jaundice.
2. What is it due to?
   It is due to increased hemolysis and poor hepatic uptake, conjugation and secretion of bilirubin. Activity of the enzyme UDP – glucuronyl transferase is low and also there is limited availability of UDP glucuronic acid for conjugation.
3. What are the treatments to be advised?
   – Drug: Phenobarbital can be given which will induce the synthesis of UDP glucuronyl transferase
   – Blood transfusion can be given
   – Phototherapy: Bilirubin can absorb blue light (420–470 nm). Exposure of the jaundiced child to blue light will convert unconjugated bilirubin into non-toxic lumirubin, which can be excreted by the kidneys.

## 2. Hemolytic Jaundice

**Case:** A second child born to Rh incompatible parents developed jaundice on the 2nd day of delivery. Child was admitted in the neonatal ICU and phototherapy was given. History revealed that the first child of the couple had no such problems during delivery. This child's blood showed increased level of total bilirubin and unconjugated bilirubin.

1. What is this due to?
   This is due to incompatibility between maternal and fetal blood groups as both the parents had Rh incompatibility. Usually the first child always escapes. But during the II pregnancy the Rh antibodies will pass from mother to fetus and they will destroy the fetal red cells even before birth, causing hemolysis.
2. What are the complications of this case?
   Increased toxic unconjugated bilirubin enters the brain as the blood-brain barrier is not fully matured and deposited in the child's brain causing kernicterus.

3. What are the treatments advised?
   Phototherapy with blue light (440 nm wavelength) isomerizes the insoluble bilirubin to more soluble isomers, which can be excreted through urine.
4. Markers of hemolytic jaundice (unconjugated hyperbilirubinemia) (prehepatic jaundice).
   a. Increased level of serum unconjugated bilirubin
   b. Increased excretion of urobilinogen
   c. Dark brown color feces due to increased level of stercobilinogen.

### 3. Hepatic Jaundice

**Case: 17 years old college student residing in hostel developed fever, nausea and vomiting for the past 3 days. He attended the medical OP and was found to be jaundiced and passing high colored urine.**

1. What is the probable diagnosis of the case?
   Hepatocellular jaundice (hepatic jaundice).
2. What will be the cause?
   May be due to viral hepatitis, which may lead to damage to parenchymal cells of liver. This affects the uptake and conjugation of bilirubin by liver cells.
3. What are the biochemical changes observed in this patient?
   - Both conjugated and unconjugated bilirubin are increased in serum.
   - Excessive excretion of bilirubin and urobilinogen in urine causes dark yellow coloured urine.
   - Increased level of serum alanine transaminase (ALT), aspartate transaminase (AST) and alkaline phosphatase (ALP).
4. What are the other causes of hepatic jaundice?
   - Alcoholic liver cirrhosis
   - Hepatocellular carcinoma
   - Toxic hepatitis due to hepatotoxic drugs and chemicals.

### 4. Obstructive Jaundice

**Case: A 40 years old fatty lady has got fever, loss of appetite and itching all over the body and also has pain over the right hypochondrium for the past one week. She is passing clay colored stools and dark colored urine for the past 3 days. Her investigation results are given below.**

- Serum total bilirubin: 8 mg%
- Conjugated bilirubin: 6.8 mg%
- Serum aspartate transaminase (AST): 180 units/L
- Serum alanine transaminase (ALT): 250 units /L
- Serum alkaline phosphatase: 90 KA units
- Urine: Bile salts ++, bile pigments++
- Urine: Urobilinogen – Negative

1. What is your probable diagnosis?
   Obstructive jaundice—probably due to gallstones.
2. What are the other causes of obstructive jaundice?
   - Stricture of bile duct
   - Cancer head of pancreas pressing over biliary system
   - Enlarged lymph nodes pressing over the bile duct.

3. Why is there clay colored stools?
   Due to the absence of stercobilinogen.
4. What is the reason for increased level of alkaline phosphatase?
   The obstruction of bile duct induces the synthesis of alkaline phosphatase enzyme by the epithelial cells of biliary tract.
5. What are the markers of obstructive jaundice?
   - Conjugated bilirubin—elevated
   - Alkaline phosphatase level—increased
   - Clay coloured stools due to the absence of stercobilinogen.

## C. Disorders of Acid-Base Balance

### 1. Metabolic Acidosis

An elderly man with poor control of diabetic was brought to the hospital with edema legs. He was found to be comatose and had rapid breathing.

**His laboratory reports are given below.**
- Blood pH: 7.2
- Serum bicarbonate: 14 mEq/L
- $pCO_2$: 30 mm of Hg
- Blood urea: 124 mg/dL
- Serum creatinine: 4.2 mg/dL
- Blood sugar: 320 mg/dL

1. Comment on the acid-base disturbance here.
   Metabolic acidosis.
2. What is your probable cause?
   Diabetes mellitus with renal failure.
3. What is normal pH?
   - Normal blood pH is between 7.38–7.42. (7.4).
4. Name the mechanisms maintaining pH.
   - Buffers of body fluids – First line of defense
   - Respiratory mechanism – Second line of defense
   - Renal mechanism – Third line of defense factors that regulate pH.
5. What is metabolic acidosis? Give the causes of metabolic acidosis.
   - It is one of the acid-base disorders.
   - Primary change is decrease in plasma bicarbonate concentration which is compensated by ↓$pCO_2$ by hyperventilation.
   - This occurs in diabetic ketoacidosis, lactic acidosis, renal failure and renal tubular acidosis.

### 2. Metabolic Alkalosis

Following surgery for intestinal obstruction a patient had continuous nasogastric aspiration for 2 days. Arterial blood gas analysis done and the results are:
- Blood pH: 7.54
- $pCO_2$: 52 mm of Hg
- Plasma bicarbonate: 32 mEq/L
- Serum sodium: 128 mEq/L

- **Serum potassium: 2.4 mEq/L**
- **Serum chloride: 96 mEq/L**

1. What is your probable diagnosis?
   Metabolic alkalosis.
2. What is it due to and what are the causes for this condition?
   - Primary change is excess of bicarbonate which is compensated by increased $pCO_2$ by hypoventilation.
   - This is seen in vomiting, diuretic therapy. Severe hypokalemia.

### 3. Respiratory Acidosis

A patient was brought to the emergency ward in a drowsy state with history of sleeping tablets poisoning. On examination he had sluggish respiration with respiratory rate of 6/min.

**His arterial blood gas report is as follows:**
- **pH: 7.2**
- **Bicarbonate: 30 mEq/L**
- **$pCO_2$: 78 mm Hg**

1. What is your probable diagnosis?
   Respiratory acidosis.
2. What is it due to?
   In respiratory acidosis, there will be primary excess of carbonic acid with increased $pCO_2$. This is compensated by increase in bicarbonate.
3. What are the other causes for this sort of condition?
   This occurs in chronic obstructive lung diseases, asthma, emphysema, paralysis of respiratory muscles, respiratory depressant toxic drugs.

### 4. Respiratory Alkalosis

A student was brought from the examination hall to the casualty with complaints of tightness of chest and hurried respiration. On examination his BP was 100/70 mm of Hg; Pulse rate 100/min.

**His ABG reports are:**
- **Blood pH: 7.52**
- **Plasma bicarbonate: 20 mEq/L**
- **$pCO_2$: 20 mm Hg**

1. What is your probable diagnosis?
   Respiratory alkalosis.
2. What is the cause for this condition?
   Hysterical hyperventilation.
3. What is respiratory alkalosis? In which conditions will it occur?
   - This is characterized by primary deficit of $pCO_2$ (Carbonic acid) which is compensated by decrease in bicarbonate.
   - This is seen in high altitude, hyperventilation (hysterical), septicemia, pregnancy, liver failure.

## D. Cardiac Disease: Myocardial Infarction

A chronic smoker aged 52 years was rushed to the hospital emergency ward from his workspot with profuse sweating, breathlessness and severe chest pain. Urgent ECG was taken and it showed the evidences of acute myocardial infarction.

O/E: Conscious.
Extremities were cold and clammy
Blood pressure: 94/60 mm Hg;
Pulse rate: 110/min; Feeble
Respiratory rate: 22/min

*Laboratory Reports*

Blood analysis

- Glucose: 140 mg%
- Urea: 28 mg%
- Total cholesterol: 280 mg%
- LDL cholesterol: 38 mg%
- Triglycerides: 400 mg%
- **Enzyme pattern in serum was called for.**
1. What were the enzymes which are elevated in this condition?
   - Enzymes elevated in myocardial infarction are creatine kinase, aspartate transaminase, lactate dehydrogenase.
   - Creatine kinase: CK MB is the first enzyme to be elevated in MI. It is released into the circulation within 6–8 hrs, reaches its peak value within 24–30 hrs and returns to normal level by 2nd or 3rd day.
   - Aspartate transaminase: Rises sharply after CPK, and reaches a peak within 48 hours of MI. It takes 4–5 days to return to normal level.
   - Lactate dehydrogenase: LDH-1 rises from the second day after infarction, attains a peak by the 3rd or 4th day and takes about 10–15 days to reach normal level. It's the last enzyme to rise and also the last enzyme to return to normal level in MI. LDH-1 is more than LDH-2 in MI (Flipped pattern).
2. Mention important cardiac markers in myocardial infarction.
   - CK-MB: It is the **first enzyme to be elevated** in MI. It is released into the circulation within 6–8 hrs, reaches its peak value within 24–30 hrs and returns to normal level by 2nd or 3rd day
   - Myoglobin: It is an oxygen-binding heme protein—raised as early as 1-4 hours after the onset. Not specific because it is increased in injury to cardiac and skeletal muscles.
   - Troponins: They bind to calcium and regulate muscle contraction.
   - T (TnT), Troponin I (TnI): TnI is specific for myocardium and not for skeletal muscles. Increased within 4–10 hours after the onset; Reached peak at 12–48 hours; The level is elevated for 4–10 days.
3. What are isoenzymes? Give example.
   - Multiple molecular forms of an enzyme catalyzing the same reaction are isoenzymes or isozymes. E.g. Lactate dehydrogenase-5-isoenzymes (LDH 1, 2, 3, 4 and 5), creatine kinase- 3 isoenzymes-(CK -1, 2, 3) and alkaline phosphatase.
   - They are physically distinct forms of the same enzyme activity.

## E. Renal Diseases

### 1. Nephrotic Syndrome

A 12-year-old boy presented with complaints of puffiness of face and swelling of legs for the past three days. On examination blood pressure was low normal. Laboratory findings are given below.
- Blood urea: 28.0 mg%
- Serum creatinine: 0.6 mg%
- Serum cholesterol: 480.0 mg
- Total protein: 4.3 g%
- Serum albumin: 1.2 g%
- Globulin: 3.3 g%
- Urine protein: 3.5 g/24 hours.
- Serum electrophoresis was done.

1. What is your probable diagnosis?
   Nephrotic syndrome.
2. What are the three important characteristics of this condition?
   Proteinuria, Hypoalbuminemia, Hypercholesterolemia.
3. Mention two important causes for this disease.
   Autoimmune disease and primary glomerular disease.
4. Give the serum electrophoretic pattern of this case
   Nephrotic syndrome - EPP is characterized by -  Albumin – reduced
   $\alpha_2$ globulin – markedly increased

### 2. Chronic Kidney Disease

An elderly male, who had a long history of high blood pressure, was brought to the hospital in a drowsy state. Biochemical investigations revealed the following:
- Blood urea: 124 mg%
- Serum creatinine: 6.8 mg%
- Serum uric acid: 8.8 mg%
- Serum inorganic phosphorus: 6.2 mg%

1. What is the probable diagnosis?
   Chronic kidney disease (CKD).
2. What is the normal urinary output per day
   Normal urine: 800–2000 mL/day. Day output is greater than night output.
3. What is meant by oliguria? Give causes.
   - **Oliguria:** Decreased volume (less than 500 mL).
   - Due to:
     - Excess of fluid loss due to vomiting, diarrhea–Dehydration
     - Acute nephritis.

4. Give the importance of creatinine clearance test.
   - Glomerulus acts as a sieve in filtering blood but it retains cells and proteins thus forming a glomerular filtrate—normally 170–180 liters/day. Out of this only 1.5 liter of fluid is excreted as urine and the rest are reabsorbed through the tubules.
   - **Glomerular filtration rate (GFR): Normal GFR is 120-125 mL/min.** This is reduced in renal failure.
   - **Clearance tests** are done to assess the glomerular filtration and renal blood flow.
   - **Renal clearance of a substance is the volume of plasma from which the substance is completely cleared by the kidney in one minute.**
   - **Clearance** = mg of substance excreted per min/mg of substance per mL of plasma; $C = U \times V/P$   $C$ = Clearance of the substance; $U$ = Concentration of the substance in urine; $P$ = Concentration of the substance in plasma; $V$ = Volume of urine passed per minute.
   - Clearance is expressed as milliliter of plasma per unit time.
   - Clearance test is done by using either endogenous markers such as urea or creatinine or exogenous markers like Inulin, $^{51}$Cr- labelled EDTA, 99Tec- labelled EDTA, etc. Out of all, creatinine clearance test is the best.
   - Creatinine clearance test is based on the rate of excretion of metabolically produced creatinine which is excreted through urine. Creatinine is freely filtered by the glomeruli but not reabsorbed by the tubules. A small amount of creatinine is secreted by the tubules.
   - 24 hours urine is collected and blood is also collected for estimation of creatinine. Urinary volume is measured (V) and the concentration of creatinine in urine (U) and plasma (P) are estimated and by using the formula $C = U \times V/P$ the creatinine clearance is calculated.
   - Normal range for creatinine clearance is 90–129 mL/min
   - Reduced creatinine clearance indicates chronic renal damage and reduced blood flow to glomeruli.
   - Normal urea clearance: 75 mL/min.
   - Normal inulin clearance: 125 mL/min.

## F. Purine Metabolism

### Gout

A middle-aged executive developed severe pain and swelling of the first right metatarsophalangeal joint with swollen right great toe after a bout of alcohol on the previous night. There was no history of injury to the toe. He had no previous similar history.
- **He was febrile**
- **His relevant laboratory reports are given below:**
  - Blood sugar: 150 mg%
  - Blood urea: 32 mg%
  - Serum uric acid: 12.2 mg%
  - Synovial fluid analysis: Needle-shaped crystals

1. What is your probable diagnosis?
   Gout.
2. What is gout? What are its types? What are they due to?

- Uric acid is the catabolic end product of purine nucleotides. When uric acid level is increased in blood, it tends to get deposited as crystals in synovial fluid of joints leading to inflammation and acute arthritis. This disease is called Gout.
- Two types of Gout: Primary and secondary gout
    - *Primary gout*: 10% is idiopathic. Others are due to inherited disorders due to abnormalities of enzymes such as (i) Super active 5-phosphoribosyl amido transferase enzyme (ii) Abnormal PRPP synthase (iii) Salvage pathway enzyme deficiencies – HGPRT-ase partial deficiency and (iv) Glucose -6 phosphatase deficiency -Von Gierke's Disease
    - *Secondary gout*: (i) Increased production of uric acid due to increased turnover of cells as in malignancy—lymphomas, leukemia, polycythemia, psoriasis, after treatment of cancer, trauma and starvation (ii) Reduced excretion of uric acid-renal failure, thiazide diuretics, lactic acidosis and ketoacidosis.
3. What is the normal uric acid level in blood and in per day urine.
    - Normal blood level of uric acid is 2–5 mg/dL for females and 3–7 mg/dL for males
    - Normal urinary excretion of uric acid is 500–700 mg/day.

# II. DEFICIENCY DISORDERS

## 1. Vitamin A Deficiency

### Night Blindness (Nyctalopia)

**Case:** A 10 years old boy has been brought to the ophthalmic clinic with complaints of poor vision during evening and night hours. On examination he was having dry and rough skin and had dryness of cornea and conjunctiva of both eyes. He belonged to a poor income group.

1. What is your probable diagnosis?
   Night blindness (Nyctalopia).
2. What is it due to?
   Due to the deficiency of vitamin A which is a fat-soluble vitamin.
3. What are the sources of vitamin A?
   **Animal:** Milk, butter, cream, cheese, egg yolk and liver, fish liver oils (Cod and shark liver oils)
   **Plant:** From its precursor beta ($\beta$) carotene which is present in papaya, carrot, mango and tomato.
4. What are the various forms of vitamin A?
   Retinal (Aldehyde), Retinol (Alcohol) and Retinoic acid (Acid).
5. What are their functions?
   A. Retinaldehyde: Vision
   B. Retinol: Reproduction
   C. Retinoic acid: Regulation of gene expression and differentiation of tissues and growth
   D. Beta carotene: Antioxidant property.
6. Who found out the visual cycle?
   George Wald.
7. What is provitamin A?
   Beta carotene—an antioxidant
8. How is vitamin A transported in blood?
   By retinol-binding protein (RBP).

9. **What are rods? What is rhodopsin? What is dark adaptation and time?**
   Retina of the eye contains the visual pigments rods and cones. Rods are responsible for perception of dim light. Rods contain Rhodopsin which is made up to 11-cis retinal and opsin (Protein).
   Bright light depletes the stores of rhodopsin in rods. So when we enter into a dark room, we cannot see anything for few minutes and after some time, there will be improvement of vision due to resynthesis of Rhodopsin. This period is called as dark adaptation time. It is increased in Vitamin A deficiency.

## 2. Vitamin D Deficiency

### Rickets

**Case: A five-year-old male child was brought to the pediatric outpatient department with deformity of bones like bow legs and knock knee. His mother reported that he started walking only after his second year of life. He looked malnourished and thin. He also had pigeon chest and beading of ribs. His laboratory report revealed decreased level of calcium and phosphorus in blood.**

1. What is your probable diagnosis?
   Rickets.
2. What is it due to?
   Due to the deficiency of vitamin D.
3. What are various forms of Vitamin D?
   Vitamin D2 – Ergocalciferol (Plant source)
   Vitamin D3 – Cholecalciferol (Animal) - from skin by the action of UV rays from sunlight.
4. What is active Vitamin D? Where is it synthesized?
   Calcitriol or 1,25-dihydroxycholecalciferol—synthesized in kidney.
5. What are the main functions of active vitamin D?
   A. It helps in absorption of calcium and phosphorus from the intestine.
   B. It increases the reabsorption of calcium by the renal tubules.
   C. It increases the mineralization of bones.
6. What are the sources of Vitamin D?
   Sunlight, fish liver oil, fish, egg yolk and milk.
7. Name the deficiency manifestation of Vitamin D in children and in adults.
   Children: Rickets. Adults: Osteomalacia.

## 3. Vitamin C Deficiency

### Scurvy

**Case: A 30-year-old lady from a village came to the dentist with the complaints of painful swollen and bleeding gums for one month duration. On examination her teeth were found to be shaky and there was loss of a tooth as well. She also had painful swelling over the left knee joint.**

1. What is your diagnosis?
   Scurvy.
2. What is it due to?
   Due to the deficiency of vitamin C (Ascorbic acid).

3. Why was there bleeding in the gums?
   Vitamin C is essential for the synthesis of collagen by acting as a cofactor for hydroxylation of proline and lysine residues as post translational modification. So in vitamin C deficiency, there is improper production of collagen and other cement substances of capillary wall and so the capillaries become fragile and cause bleeding gums and subcutaneous hemorrhage.
4. What is the treatment for Scurvy?
   Megadoses of vitamin C (1000 mg to 5000 mg).
5. What are the sources of Vitamin C?
   Gooseberry, Citrus fruits—lime, lemon, oranges and green leafy vegetables.
6. What are the biochemical functions of vitamin C?
   A. It is needed for the post-translational hydroxylation of proline and lysine residues of collagen and strengthens collagen.
   B. It is an antioxidant.
   C. It helps in the hydroxylation reactions of tryptophan metabolism and steroid synthesis.
7. Why vitamin C cannot be synthesized in animals and human beings?
   It cannot be synthesized because of the absence of the enzyme gulonolactone oxidase in uronic acid pathway of glucose.

## 4. Vitamin $B_{12}$ Deficiency—Macrocytic Anemia

**A 50-year-old female:** Working as a daily wage earner, came to the medical outpatient department, with complaints of fatigue, numbness and tingling sensations in her extremities for the past 4 months. She is not a diabetic or hypertensive. She had regular periods.
- On examination – she is anemic; Pulse 86/mt; Tongue – beefy red in color
- Neurological examination revealed numbness and decreased vibration senses in the extremities. Her
- Hb-6.0 g/dL
- Peripheral blood smear shows macrocytic megaloblastic red blood cells

1. What is the probable diagnosis of this patient?
   Macrocytic anemia.
2. What is the most likely cause for this case?
   Vitamin $B_{12}$ deficiency.
3. What are the sources and daily requirements of this nutrient?
   Sources: Only animal sources -liver, curds and intestinal bacteria.
   Daily requirement: 1-2 microgram.
4. Give any two biochemical functions of the nutrient.
   a. Methyl cobalamin: Prevents folate trap. Transmethylation of homocysteine to methionine.
   b. Deoxyadenosylcobalamin: Isomerization of methylmalonyl-CoA to succinyl-CoA.

## 5. Protein-Energy Malnutrition (PEM)

### Kwashiorkor

**Case:** A 3-year-old plumpy male child was brought to the outpatient department by the parents with swelling on the face and all over the body, distension of abdomen, sparse hair, peeling of skin in the swollen areas for 2 months. They also complained that the child had watery diarrhea and cough for the past one week. Parents are daily workers with very poor income having 3 children. This boy was the second child and he had one elder sister of 5 years old and a younger brother of 3 months old. This boy was given a diet of rice *kanji* which was mainly of carbohydrates. No cereals or milk were given. The investigation reports are given below.

### Blood

- Total WBC count: 8600 cells/cu.mm.
- Differential count: P70%, L26%, E3%, M1%
- Hb: 9 g%
- RBC count: 4.1 million/cumm
- Total protein: 3.5 g/dL
- Serum albumin: 1.5 g/dL
- (F) blood glucose: 60 mg/dL
- Blood urea: 18 mg/dL
- Serum potassium: 2.8 mEq/L

### Urine

- Albumin: Negative
- Sugar: Negative

1. What is your probable diagnosis?
   Protein-energy malnutrition—Kwashiorkor.
2. Why is there swelling of the body?
   Hypoproteinemia and hypoalbuminemia lower the colloid osmotic pressure causing the movement of fluid into the interstitial compartment causing swelling.
3. How does Kwashiorkor differ from Marasmus?
   Marasmus is mainly due to the deficiency of calorie only whereas Kwashiorkor is due to protein deficiency. Edema will be absent in Marasmus and the skin will be dry and no change in hair. Serum albumin will be around 2 to 3 g/dL and serum cortisol will be increased.
4. How will you treat Marasmus and Kwashiorkor?
   Parents should be advised to prepare hygienic good quality and economical protein diet such as cereals, soyabean, Bengal gram or peanuts along with milk. (3 parts of vegetable proteins + 1 part of milk protein). Child should be given proper attention by the parents and should not be neglected.

## ■ III. INHERITED DISORDERS (INBORN ERRORS OF METABOLISM)

## A. Carbohydrate Metabolism

### 1. Lactose Intolerance

Case: A black person aged 16 years, came to the casualty in the morning with vomiting and diarrhea and flatulence. He did not have fever or jaundice. He reported that these symptoms occurred after a party in which he consumed large quantities of ice creams. He had the same symptoms 2 months back after taking lots of milk sweets.

1. What is your provisional diagnosis in the case?
   Lactose intolerance.

2. What is it due to?
   Deficiency of the enzyme lactase (β-galactosidase) due to reduced production. As the lactose in the ice cream was not digested there were symptoms of abdominal discomfort and diarrhea.
3. How will you treat these cases?
   Patient should be advised to stop taking dairy products.
   Curd or yogurt can be given which contains β-galactosidase enzyme. β-Galactosidase is also present in yeast. Commercial preparation of β-galactosidase is also available.

## 2. Galactosemia

**Case: A newborn baby with jaundice was examined by a child specialist at a neonatal ward and was found to have enlarged liver and cataract in both the eyes.**

Urine gave positive result for reducing sugar with Benedict's reagent. Blood investigations revealed a very low glucose in blood and high levels of unconjugated bilirubin. The child specialist advised to stop feeding the baby with milk and instead glucose solution was given orally. The child started improving:

1. What is your diagnosis?
   Galactosemia.
2. What is it due to?
   Mainly due to the deficiency of the enzyme galactose 1 phosphate uridyl transferase. It may be also due to the deficiency of galactokinase and galactose – 4-epimerase enzymes.
3. What are the basis of the biochemical changes that occur which lead to all the symptoms?
   A. Galactose accumulates in the cell and it is then reduced by aldose reductase enzyme to produce dulcitol. Due to the osmotic effect dulcitol in the lens produces cataract.
   B. Increased galactose will inhibit galactokinase and glycogen phosphorylase to produce hypoglycemia.
   C. Uptake of bilirubin in liver is reduced and also resulting in reduced conjugation of bilirubin which leads to unconjugated hyperbilirubinemia.
   D. Generalized aminoaciduria may occur due to accumulation of galactose 1- P in the renal tubules.
4. What are the treatments to be suggested?
   To stop feeding of milk and to give galactose free diet to prevent brain damage. Cataract can be corrected by surgery.

## 3. Hereditary Fructose Intolerance (HFI)

**Case: A 9 months old child was brought to the pediatrician with a history of vomiting, night sweats and tremors. History from the mother revealed that the baby was weaned off breast milk since one week and she was giving him plenty of fruit juice along with cow's milk. There was mild enlargement of liver.**

**Urine of the baby gave positive result for reducing sugar – Benedict's test. But the blood glucose was only 50 mg%.**

1. What is your probable diagnosis?
   Hereditary fructose intolerance.
2. What is it due to?
   Due to the deficiency of the enzyme aldolase B.

3. Why is the blood glucose low?
   Due to the absence of aldolase B, fructose 1 phosphate accumulates and this will inhibit glycogen phosphorylase which leads to deposition of glycogen in liver and causes hypoglycemia.
4. How will you confirm the diagnosis?
   Positive Benedict's test shows presence of reducing sugar, positive Seliwanoff's test- confirmatory test for fructose, chromatography of urine for sugars, restriction fragment length polymorphism.

## B. Lipid Metabolism

### Familial Hypercholesterolemia (FHC)

Case: A boy aged 9 years came to the outpatient department with cutaneous xanthoma on the elbow and hands. His father had expired at the age of 35 years following a sudden heart attack.

The investigations done for the boy revealed the following results:
- Urine: Albumin, Sugar: Negative
- Blood glucose (Fasting): 80 mg%
- Total cholesterol: 525 mg%
- LDL cholesterol: 360 mg%
- HDL cholesterol: 22 mg%
- Triglycerides: 120 mg%

1. What is your probable diagnosis?
   Familial hypercholesterolemia (FHC) Type IIa hyperlipoproteinemia (Frederickson classification).
2. What is it due to?
   Due to defect in LDL receptors.
3. What are its consequences if not treated?
   The boy may develop premature atherosclerosis which can lead to myocardial infarction and early death.
4. What are the treatments to be suggested?
   - To take low cholesterol diet
   - To take more PUFA and cholesterol reducing drugs.
   - To consult cardiologist and evaluate the cardiac condition.
5. Name some hypolipidemic drugs:
   a. HMG COA reductase inhibitors – (Statins): Atorvastatin, Simvastatin
   b. Bile acid-binding resins: Cholestyramine, colestipol
   c. Probucol: Prevents LDL accumulation
   d. Nicotinic acid: Inhibits lipolysis
   e. Aspirin: Antiplatelet drug
   f. Antioxidants: Vitamin E.

## C. Amino Acid Metabolism

### 1. Homocystinuria

Case: A 6-year-old child with delayed milestones was reported to have posterior dislocation of the lens in the right eye. The child was having poor intelligence and also waddling gait.
1. What is your probable diagnosis?
   Homocystinuria - Classical (Type I).

2. What is the biochemical defect and what are the various types of homocystinuria?
   - Type I (Classical) – deficiency of Cystathionine beta synthase enzyme (PLP dependent) in methionine metabolism
   - Type II: Deficiency of N5,N10-Methylenetetrahydrofolate reductase (Folic acid/$B_{12}$ metabolism)
   - Type III: Cobalamin deficiency (Methylcobalamin)
   - Type IV: Defective intestinal absorption of $B_{12}$.
3. What are the clinical and laboratory findings?
   - General symptoms: Mental retardation
   - Charlie Chaplin gait
   - Skeletal deformity due to osteoporosis
   - Ectopia lentis (Subluxation of lens)
   - Myopia, Glaucoma
   - Signs of intravascular thrombosis.

   **Laboratory Findings:**
   Urine: Increased level of methionine and homocysteine (>300 mg/day) Positive cyanide nitroprusside test.
   Blood plasma: Increased homocysteine (>100 mm/L) and cysteine—reduced.
4. What is the treatment suggested?
   Diet low in methionine and rich in cysteine, Vitamin $B_6$ and folic acid to be supplemented.

## 2. Phenylketonuria (PKU)

**Case: A 1-year-old boy child with delayed milestones and lethargy, was brought to the children's OP with complaints of tremors and fits. Child was not able to respond to the questions asked. There were few hypopigmented patches around the body and also the child smelt mousy body odor.**

1. What is your probable diagnosis?
   Phenylketonuria (PKU) – Autosomal recessive (AR).
2. What are its types and causes?
   - Type I: Classical – deficiency of phenylalanine hydroxylase
   - Type II, III: Deficiency of dihydrobiopterin reductase
   - Type IV, V: Deficiency of enzymes synthesizing biopterin.
3. What are the biochemical and clinical manifestations?
   Biochemical changes:
   - Accumulation of phenylalanine leading to high levels of phenylalanine in blood by Tandem mass spectrometry (>20 mg/dL)
   - Urine—increased levels of phenyl pyruvate, lactate and acetate
   - Rapid screening test— Guthrie test
   - Ferric chloride test—in urine
   - DNA probes to detect defective phenylalanine hydroxylase and other enzymes.
   Clinical findings:
   - Mental retardation—Low IQ
   - Agitation, tremors, convulsions
   - Hypopigmented patches
   - Mousy body odor—due to increased level of phenyl lactate in sweat.

4. What is the treatment?
   - Early detection to prevent mental retardation
   - Advised to give diet low in phenylalanine (Tapioca- advisable).

### *3. Alkaptonuria*

**Case: A mother brought her one year old child to the pediatrician, with the complaints that the diaper of the baby becomes black on urination though the urine passed by the child looked clear. The parents are first degree consanguineous couple. The other two siblings were normal. Growth and intelligence of the child was also normal.**

1. What is your probable diagnosis? What is it due to?
   Alkaptonuria—due to the deficiency of the enzyme homogentisate oxidase in tyrosine metabolism, resulting in excretion of homogentisate in urine.
2. Why did the diaper changes into black in color?
   The excreted homogentisate is oxidized and polymerized to black colored alkaptone bodies on exposure to air.
3. What are the later complications of the condition?
   Ochronosis—occurs around 30–40 years. It the deposition of alkaptone bodies in the intervertebral disks, cartilages of nose and pinna of ear. Deposition in the joint cavities causing arthritis.
4. How will you diagnose this condition?
   - Blackening of urine on standing.
   - Positive ferric chloride test.
   - Benedict's test: Positive, due to reducing activity of homogentisate.
5. Is there any treatment to be given?
   No specific treatment
   Low protein diet with less phenylalanine to be recommended.

## ■ IV. HORMONAL DISORDERS

## A. Thyroid Disorder

### *1. Hypothyroidism*

**Case: A 40-year-old obese lady came with the complaints of lethargy, hoarseness of voice, constipation for the past four months. During winters she felt increased cold sensitivity. On examination, she had coarse skin and her pulse rate was 62 per minute. The results of the relevant investigations are as follows:**

- **Hb: 8.4 g%**
- **Serum: $T_3$, $T_4$ levels decreased, TSH level increased**
- **Serum cholesterol 340 mg/dL**
- **ECG showing low heart rate and low voltage complexes.**

1. What is the probable diagnosis?
   Hypothyroidism.
2. What is it due to? How can you correlate the changes seen?
   Hypothyroidism occurs due to the disease of thyroid gland which leads to decreased levels of the thyroid hormones. Hence thyroid stimulating hormone (TSH) secretion by the pituitary is increased.

3. What are the possible diseases of thyroid gland which can cause hypothyroidism?
   A. Autoimmune thyroiditis
   B. Thyroidectomy
   C. Drugs like lithium.
4. What is the treatment for hypothyroidism?
   Replacement by oral preparation; Tab. Thyroxine 50 to 200 µg/day.

## B. Parathyroid Disorder

### 2. Hyperparathyroidism

**Case:** A 50-year-old lady gives history of lethargy, depression, muscle weakness and poor appetite for the past six months. She also had episodes of renal colic and was found to have renal stones earlier. The results of the relevant investigations are given below.
- **Serum calcium: 12 mg/dL**
- **Serum phosphate: 2 mg/dL**
- **Serum alkaline phosphatase: 230 units/L**

1. What is the probable diagnosis?
   Hyperparathyroidism.
2. What test can be done to confirm your diagnosis?
   Serum level of parathyroid hormone (PTH) increased.
3. What is the cause of this disease?
   Parathyroid adenoma.
4. How can we treat this disease?
   High fluid intake
   Treatment for renal stones
   May require surgical removal of adenoma.

# SECTION 8
# Objective Structured Practical Examination

## Section Outline

44. Objective Structured Practical Examination

# CHAPTER 44

# Objective Structured Practical Examination

## ■ OBJECTIVE STRUCTURED PRACTICAL EXAMINATION (OSPE)

Objective structured practical examination (OSPE) simply known as on the spot practical examination has been recommended by the Medical Council of India and many universities have already started doing it as a part of practical syllabus. OSPE is a checklist of all the steps involved in a particular practical test. These steps are objective which will be observed by the teacher/examiner and evaluation will be done on all the steps performed in the serial order by the student. Here the teacher/examiner will be simply observing the steps without any interference. At the end, one or two relevant question(s) may be asked to the students. Marks will be allotted for the performance and also for answering the questions.

OSPE will be conducted in a performance station. A suitable command to perform a particular test will be kept on the table (For example: Perform Benedict's test with the given solution). One or two relevant question(s) can be added to the chart for which the student has to give answers. Marks are allotted for each step and for the questions. Reagents for the particular test can be mixed with some other reagents and kept on the nearby rack. The solution to be tested is kept in a beaker or a bottle and labelled. Necessary pipettes should be kept over the table in the rack. If heating is needed, the burner should be kept ready with match box. A mark sheet with divisions for each step can be prepared and kept ready.

About 2-3 stations can be kept as **'Performance stations'** where the examiner can sit and watch or observe what the student is doing without asking any questions till the student completes the work. Relevant questions can be asked at the end to know how the student understands about the principle and importance of the test.

Let us see the example of performing Benedict's test.

## Comment and Questions

Perform Benedict's test in the given solution.
1. What is your observation? What is the color of the precipitate?
2. Depending upon the color, what is your inference?
3. If the color is green/yellow/orange, what would be the level of glucose in the urine?
4. What is the purpose of this test?
5. What are the compositions of Benedict's reagent?
6. Why glucose is a reducing sugar?

## Model Evaluation Sheet

- Take a clean dry test tube: 1 mark
- Pipette out exactly 5 mL of Benedict's reagent: 1 mark
- Add 8 drops of urine and mix thoroughly: 1 mark
- Fix the test tube in a test tube holder
- Light the Bunsen burner and boil for 2 minutes: 1 mark
- Cool it under the tap water: 1 mark

**Questions:** 5 marks

Other tests which can be asked under OSPE:
A. Test for carbohydrates
   1. Benedict's test—for reducing sugars
   2. Molisch's test—for carbohydrates
   3. Seliwanoff's test—for fructose
   4. Iodine test—for starch
B. Test for proteins/Amino acids
   1. Biuret test
   2. Sulphosalicylic acid
   3. Heat coagulation test
   4. Heller's test
C. Other tests (Abnormal urine)
   1. Hay's test for bile salts
   2. Rothera's test for ketone bodies
   3. Benzidine test for blood.

Quantitative tests can also be monitored under OSPE and scores will be given separately for deproteinization, mixing various reagents in the particular quantity, mode of heating in water bath/time given for color to be developed, and also taking readings from colorimeter—setting up the appropriate wavelength/taking up the cuvette/taking readings for blank, standard and test separately.

# SECTION 9

# Reagents

## Section Outline

45. Reagent Preparation

# CHAPTER 45

# Reagent Preparation

## ■ PREPARATION OF REAGENTS (FOR THE USE OF THE LABORATORY)

### I. Test for Carbohydrates

1. **Molisch's reagent**
   Dissolve 1 gram α-naphthol in 100 mL of 95% ethanol.
2. **Seliwanoff's reagent – For Fructose**
   Dissolve 50 mg resorcinol in 33 mL of concentrated hydrochloric acid and dilute to 100 mL with water.
3. **Bial's reagent – For Pentoses**
   Dissolve 300 mg of orcinol in 100 mL of concentrated hydrochloric acid and add 5 drops of 10% ferric chloride solution (Dilute solution of orcinol in 30% hydrochloric acid).
4. **Benedict's qualitative reagent**
   Dissolve 173 g of sodium citrate and 100 g of anhydrous sodium carbonate in 600 mL of water with the aid of heat in a beaker. In another beaker dissolve 17.3 g of copper sulfate ($CuSO_4.5H_2O$) in 100 mL of water and add this to the first beaker slowly with constant stirring. Make up to one litre with water in one litre flask.
5. **N/50 Iodine solution: For starch**
   Dilute 10 mL of 0.1 N iodine to 500 mL with 2% potassium iodide.

### II. Test for Proteins

1. **Biuret reagent**
   Dissolve 45 g of sodium potassium tartrate (Rochelle salt) in 400 mL of 0.2 N NaOH and add 15 g of $CuSO_4.5H_2O$ and stir to get a complete solution. Add 5 g of potassium iodide and dissolve. Make up to 1 litre with 0.2 NaOH.
   Dilute 200 mL of stock solution of Biuret reagent and make up to 1 litre with 0.2 N NaOH which contains 5 g of Potassium iodide per litre.
2. **Ninhydrin reagent (0.2 %)**
   Dissolve 2 g of ninhydrin in one litre of distilled water.
3. **Millon's reagent**
   Dissolve 10 g of mercuric sulfate in 50 mL of water and add 10 mL conc. $H_2SO_4$ and make volume to 100 mL with distilled water.
4. **Sodium Nitrite (1%)**
   Dissolve 1 g of sodium nitrite in 100 mL of distilled water.

5. **Sulphanilic acid (0.5% in 2% HCl)**
   Dissolve 500 mg of sulphanilic acid in 100 mL of 2% HCl (6 mL of conc. HCl in 100 mL of distilled water).
6. **Formalin solution (1 in 500)**
   Add 1 mL of formalin in 500 mL of distilled water.
7. **Mercuric sulfate (10%)**
   Dissolve 10 g of mercuric sulphate in 100 mL of distilled water.

## III. Test for Non-protein Nitrogenous Substances: Normal Urine

1. **Sodium hypobromite reagent**
   Add 25 mL of liquid bromine in 250 mL of 40% NaOH. Cool during mixing (To be prepared freshly).
2. **Urease suspension**
   10 g of Horse Gram powder is mixed with 100 mL of 30% ethanol.
3. **Benedict's uric acid reagent**
   Dissolve 100 g of pure sodium tungstate in a 1 litre flask with 600 mL of water. Add 50 g of arsenic acid ($As_2O_5$) and 25 mL of 85% phosphoric acid and 20 mL of conc. HCl. Boil for 20 minutes, cool and dilute to one litre.

## IV. Analysis of Gastric Juice and Bile

1. **Gastric juice (artificial)**
   Mix 300 mL of 0.1 N NaOH and 0.68 g of $KH_2PO_4$ and make up to volume with water. This solution gives both free and total acidity in normal range.
2. **Topfer's indicator**
   Dissolve 0.5 g dimethylaminoazobenzene in 100 mL of 95% ethanol.
3. **Fouchet's reagent**
   Dissolve 25 g of trichloroacetic acid in 50 mL of water. Add 10 mL of 10% ferric chloride and make up to 100 mL with water.
4. **Uffleman's reagent**
   To 1% aqueous phenol, add a solution of 10% ferric chloride solution dropwise until a blue colour is developed. Prepare freshly.

## V. Test for Normal Urine

1. **Phenolphthalein indicator**
   Dissolve 200 mg of phenolphthalein in 100 mL of ethanol.
2. **Ehrlich's reagent**
   Dissolve 250 g of dimethyl amino benzaldehyde in 150 mL of conc. HCl and make the volume to one litre with distilled water.

## VI. Test for Abnormal Urine

1. **Sulfosalicylic acid (20%)**
   Dissolve 20 g of sulfosalicylic acid in 100 mL of distilled water.
2. **Rothera's mixture:**
   Mix the crushed sodium nitroprusside crystals and ammonium sulfate in the ratio of 1:2 (w/w).

## VII: CSF Analysis

**Pandy's reagent:** Dissolve 10 gm of phenol in 150 mL of distilled water to get a clear, colorless solution.

## ■ QUANTITATIVE ESTIMATIONS

## I. Blood Glucose

### A. Folin Wu Method

1. **Sodium Tungstate—10%:**
   Dissolve 10 g of sodium tungstate in 100 mL of distilled water.
2. **2/3N Sulphuric acid:**
   Dilute 18.5 mL of conc. Sulphuric acid to one litre with distilled water.
3. **Alkaline copper reagent:**
   a. Dissolve 24 g of anhydrous sodium carbonate and 12 g of sodium potassium tartrate (Rochelle salt) in 250 mL of distilled water. Add with stirring 4 g of copper sulphate ($CuSO_4.5H_2O$) in 50 mL of water followed by 16 g of sodium bicarbonate.
   b. Separately dissolve 180 g of anhydrous sodium sulphate in 500 mL water, boil and cool.
   c. Mix the two solutions and make it up to one litre with distilled water.
4. **Phosphomolybdic acid reagent:**
   Dissolve 35 g of molybdic acid and 5 g of sodium tungstate in 200 mL of 10% NaOH in one litre beaker. Add 200 mL water and boil till all ammonia from the molybdic acid is removed (Test by phenolphthalein taken at the tip of the glass rod) and cool. Transfer to a 500 mL flask with washings and dilute to about 350 mL with distilled water. Add 125 mL of 85% phosphoric acid and make up to 500 mL and mix.
5. **Standard glucose-stock—1 g%:**
   Dissolve 1 g of glucose in 100 mL of 0.25% benzoic acid solution.
6. **Benzoic acid (0.25%):**
   Dissolve 2.5 g of benzoic acid in 100 mL of water. Warm to dissolve and make up to one litre with distilled water.

### B. O-Toluidine Method

7. **O-Toluidine reagent:**
   To 5 g of thiourea, add 90 mL of O-Toluidine and dilute to one litre with glacial acetic acid. Store in a brown amber bottle and keep the reagent in refrigerator.
8. **Glucose standard (O-T method):**
   Dissolve 10 mg of glucose in 50 mL distilled water. Add 30 mL of 10% trichloroacetic acid. Make up the volume to 100 mL with distilled water.

## II. Urea Estimation

### Diacetyl Monoxime (DAM) Method

1. **Diacetyl monoxime/Thiosemicarbazide (Dam/TSC) reagent (coloring reagent):**
   Mix 67 mL each of diacetyl monoxime (2.5 g% in distilled water) and thiosemicarbazide (0.5 g% in water) in water. Make final volume to one litre with water.

2. **Acid reagent:**
   Add 1.0 mL of reagent A to 1.0 L of reagent B. Mix and keep in dark bottle to refrigerator.
   *Reagent A:*
   Dissolve 5 g $FeCl_3$ in 20–50 mL of water. Transfer to a measuring cylinder. Add 100 mL of orthophosphoric acid slowly. Make the final volume to 250 mL with water.
   *Reagent B:*
   Add 200 mL of conc. $H_2SO_4$ to 800 mL of water slowly.
3. **Urea standard:**
   Dilute stock standard (100 mg%) to make a working standard of 1 mg% with water.

## III. Estimation of Creatinine (Alkaline Picrate Method/Jaffe's Reaction)

1. **Sodium Tungstate—10%:**
   Dissolve 10 g of sodium tungstate in 100 mL of distilled water.
2. **2/3N Sulfuric acid:**
   Dilute 18.5 mL of conc. sulfuric acid to one litre with distilled water.
3. **Saturated Picric acid in distilled water**
4. **Creatinine standard:**
   Stock (100 mg%): Dissolve 1 g of creatinine in 0.1 N HCl. (Dilute 8.66 mL of conc. HCl to one litre of water) to a final volume of one litre.
   Working (1 mg%): Dilute 1 mL of stock to 100 mL with distilled water.

## IV. Estimation of Total Protein (Biuret Method)

1. **Biuret reagent:**
   *Stock solution:*
   Dissolve 45 g of sodium potassium tartrate (Rochelle salt) in 400 mL of 0.2 N NaOH and add 15 g of $CuSO_4.5H_2O$ and stir to get a complete solution. Add 5 g of potassium iodide and dissolve. Make up to 1 litre with 0.2 NaOH.
   *Biuret reagent:*
   Dilute 200 mL of stock solution of Biuret reagent and make up to 1 litre with 0.2 N NaOH which contains 5 g of potassium iodide per litre.
2. **Protein standard:**
   Stock (1 g%)
   Dissolve 1 g bovine albumin in 100 mL of saline.
   Working standard: (5 mg/mL)
   Dilute 50 mL to 100 mL with saline

## V. Estimation of Uric Acid (Caraway Method)

1. **Phosphotungstic acid reagent:**
   *Stock:*
   Dissolve 50 g of sodium tungstate in 400 mL of water and add 40 mL of 85% phosphoric acid. Reflux for 2 hours and then cool. Make final volume to 500 mL.
   *Working:* Dilute 1 mL of stock to 10 mL with water.

2. **Tungstic acid reagent**:
   Add 50 mL of 10% sodium tungstate in 50 mL of 2/3N $H_2SO_4$ (dilute 18.3 mL of conc. $H_2SO_4$ to one litre of water) and make up the volume to 800 mL with distilled water. Add few drops of phosphoric acid and preserve.
3. **Uric acid standard:**
   *Stock*: (100 mg%)
   Add 100 mg of uric acid in 100 mL of 1% lithium carbonate. (Dissolve 1 g of lithium carbonate in 100 mL of water)
   Working (1 mg%)
   Dilute 1 mL of stock to 100 mL with water.

# SECTION 10

# Normal Values

**Section Outline**

46. Normal Values

# CHAPTER 46

# Normal Values

## Normal Levels in Biological Fluids

| S. No. | Biochemical substance | Level in serum/plasma | Level in per day urine |
|---|---|---|---|
| 1. | Bilirubin—Total | 0.2–1.1 mg% | |
| | Bilirubin—Direct | 0.1–0.4 mg% | |
| | Bilirubin—Indirect | 0.2–0.6 mg% | |
| 2. | Lipid profile | | |
| | Cholesterol—Total | 150–200 mg% | |
| | High-density cholesterol (HDL) | 30–60 mg% | |
| | Low-density cholesterol (LDL) | 80–130 mg% | |
| | Very-low-density cholesterol (VLDL) | 20–40 mg% | |
| | Triglycerides | 50–200 mg% | |
| 3. | Creatinine | 0.6–1.2 mg% | 1–2 g |
| 4. | Glucose | | — |
| | Fasting | 70–110 mg% | — |
| | Postprandial | 90–140 mg% | — |
| | Random | 80–120 mg% | |
| 5 | Hemoglobin | 13–15 g% | |
| | Glycosylated Hb (HbA1c) | 4–6.5% | — |
| 6 | Urea | 15–40 mg% | 15–30 g |
| | Blood urea nitrogen (BUN) | 8–20 mg% | — |
| 7 | Uric acid—Male | 3.5–7.0 mg% | 250–750 mg |
| | Uric acid—Female | 2.5–6.5 mg% | — |
| 8 | Protein—Total | 6.0–8.0 g% | <150 mg |
| | Albumin | 3.5–5.0 g% | |
| | Globulin | 2.5–3.5 g% | |
| | A:G ratio | 1.5:1 | |
| | Fibrinogen | 0.2–0.4 g% | |
| 9. | Inorganic substances | | |
| | 1. Calcium | 9–11 mg% | 250 mg |
| | 2. Phosphorus | 2.5 to 4.5 mg/dL | — |

*(Contd...)*

(Contd...)

| S. No. | Biochemical substance | Level in serum/plasma | Level in per day urine |
|---|---|---|---|
| | 3. Electrolytes | | |
| | ➤ Sodium | 136–145 mEq/L | — |
| | ➤ Potassium | 3.5–5 mEq/L | — |
| | ➤ Chloride | 96–106 mEq/L | 170–250 mEq/L |
| | ➤ Bicarbonate | 22–26 mEq/L | — |
| | 4. Inorganic phosphorus | 3.0–4.0 mg% | 1 g |
| | 5. Iodine | 4–10 µg% | — |
| | 6. Iron | 50–150 µg% | — |

## ■ ENZYME LEVELS (SERUM)

| | |
|---|---|
| Acid phosphatase | 2.5–12 IU/L (1–3 KA units/dL) (King Armstrong) |
| Alkaline phosphatase | 40–125 IU/L (3–13 KA units/dL) (King Armstrong) |
| Alanine transaminase (ALT/SGPT) | 13–35 IU/L |
| Aspartate transaminase (AST/SGOT) | 8–40 IU/L |
| Amylase | 50–120 IU/L (80–180 Somogyi units/dL) |
| Creatine kinase—Total | 15–100 U/L |
| Creatine kinase—MB | <5% of total CK |
| Gamma glutamyl transferase (GGT) | 10–40 IU/L |
| Lactate dehydrogenase | 100–200 IU/L |
| Lipase | 50–175 IU/L |

| *Cerebrospinal fluid* | |
|---|---|
| Protein (Mostly albumin) | 15–45 mg% |
| Glucose | 50–80 mg% |
| Chloride | 120–130 mEq/L as chloride ion |

| *Hormones* | *Serum* | *Urine* |
|---|---|---|
| Thyroid stimulating hormone (TSH) | 0.5–5 µU/mL | — |
| Thyroxine ($T_4$) | 5–12 µg/dL | — |
| Triiodothyronine ($T_3$) | 120–190 ng/dL | — |

# WORKSHEET

## Observations and Calculations

# Work sheet: Observations and Calculations

# Work sheet: Observations and Calculations

# Index

Page numbers followed by *f* refer to figure.

**A**
Absorption photometry 45
Acid 13
　accidental swallowing of 9
　acetic 106, 109
　arachidonic 160, 161
　benzoic 193
　burns 9
　dienoic 160
　linoleic 160, 161
　nucleic 94
　oleic 160
　reagent 194
Acid-base
　balance, disorders of 171
　disease 118
　disorder 68, 120, 148, 152
　disturbances 120
　　diagnosis of 119
Acidity 23
Acidosis 120
Addison's disease 57, 116
Adenine 94
Adrenal cortex 152
Adrenal function tests 152
Adrenal insufficiency, secondary 153
Adrenal medulla 152, 153
Adrenaline 153
Adrenocortical functions,
　　assessment of 153
Agglutination 123
Alanine transaminase 91
Albumin 28, 110
Albumin: globulin ratio 73, 75
Albuminuria 23, 28, 147
Alcohol 56
Alcoholism 81
Aldosteronism
　primary 153
　secondary 153
Alkaline
　copper reagent 193
　copper reduction methods 51
　hypobromite test 26

　phosphatase 92, 121
　　determination of 92
　picrate method 62, 64, 194
　sodium carbonate 96
Alkaptonuria 37, 37*f*, 183
Alumina 80
Amino acid 106
　metabolism 181
　paper chromatography of 105
　separation of 105
　specific 106
　tyrosine 153
Amino antipyrine method 92
Ammonia 24
　test for 26
Anabolic steroids 116
Antibody 123
　detection 121
Antigen
　detection 122
　enzyme-labeled 121
　specific 123
Anuria 22
Arterial blood
　gas analyzer 118
　sample 118
Aspartate aminotransferase 91
Augmented histamine test 134
Autoanalyzer 125, 125*f*
　advantages of 127
　drawbacks of 127
　method 68
　parts of 126
Automated micropipettes 8
Ayostix 68
Azobilirubin 140

**B**
Balanced diet 158
Basal gastric secretion 134
Basal metabolic rate 157
Batch analyzer 126
Beakers 7
Beer's law 45

Beer-Lambert's law 45
Benedict's qualitative
　reagent 191
　test 58
Benedict's test 28, 180
Benedict's uric acid
　reagent 192
　test 26
Benzidine test 30, 32, 134
Bial's reagent 191
Bicarbonate, fractional excretion
　　of 147
Bile
　analysis of 142, 143, 192
　duct, tumor pressing on 89
　functions of 143
　secretion, factors affecting 143
　test for 135
　　proteins in 144
Bile pigments 31, 135, 142
　test for 31, 32, 144
Bile salt 30, 135, 143
　test for 30, 32, 143
Biliary tract, stricture in 89
Biliary transport, defective 89
Bilirubin 142
　conjugated 87
　direct 88
　estimation of 87, 140
Biochemical tests, basis of 165
Biomedical wastes 10
Biuret
　method 73, 74, 194
　reagent 74, 191, 194
Blood 30, 179
　actual volume of 55, 63, 70, 96
　analyzer 119
　collection of 11
　components of 11
　gas
　　analyzer 118
　　measurements 120
　glucose 193
　　estimation of 51, 52, 54, 102

hemolysis of 11
in urine, test for 30
phosphorus in 84
sample
  tested 119
  types of 11
specimen 52
test for 32
urea
  decrease in 71
  increase in 71
Bone
  diseases 93
  metastatic carcinoma of 83
Bromocresol green method 74
Buffer 13
  capacity 13
  preparation of 13
Burns 116
Butanol 106

## C

Calcium 23, 119
Caloric requirement 157
Capillary action 106
Capillary tube 114
Caraway method 94, 194
Carbohydrate 105, 159
  metabolism 179
    congenital disorders of 35
  test for 191
Carboxypeptidase 137
Cardiac disease 173
Catecholamines, actions of 154
Centrifuges 5
Cerebrospinal fluid 19, 41, 200
  analysis of 42
  collection of 41
    lumbar puncture for 41f
  composition of 41
  normal composition of 41
Chief cells 133
Chloride 23, 117, 119
  analysis of 42
Chloroform 12
Cholestasis 93
  marker of 141
Cholesterol 79
  level, decrease in 78
  methods of estimation of 77
Chromatographic separations 39
Chromatography 105
Chymotrypsin 137
Citrate 12
Clearance tests 146
Cobalamin deficiency 39
Color, development of 63
Colorimeter 126
  parts of 46, 46f

Colorimetry
  calculation 47
  end-point analysis 48
  filters 47
  principles of 45
  procedure 47
Coloring reagent 193
Compound lipids 160
Congenital cystic kidney diseases 71
Congestive cardiac failure 116
Conical flasks 7
Conn's syndrome 153
Copper sulfate 53, 74
Corticosteroids 56
Cortisone therapy, prolonged 116
*Corynebacterium ureafaciens* 65
Creatinine 25, 63, 64
  clearance 62, 65–67
  test 146, 175
  estimation of 64, 194
    methods of 65
  picrate 63
  synthesis of 65f
  test for 27
Cretinism 151
Crigler-Najjar syndrome 89
Cushing's disease 116
Cushing's syndrome 56, 116, 117, 153
Cyanide nitroprusside test 39
Cystathionine beta synthase
  deficiency 38

## D

Deficiency disorders 166, 176
Dehydration 116, 117
Deoxyribonucleic acid
  extraction of 129
  isolation, applications of 129
Desiccators 6
Detoxification function 140
Diabetes mellitus 23, 29, 56, 59, 61f, 68, 81, 148, 152, 159, 166
  gestational 59
  diagnosis of 60
  type 1 166
  type 2 167
Diabetic ketoacidosis 120, 167
Diabetic nephropathy, indication of 147
Diacetyl monoxime 69, 193
  method 69, 70, 193
  procedure 69
  reagents 69
Dialyzer 126
Diarrhea 116, 150
Dilution tests 146
Dinitrophenylhydrazine 90
Direct colorimetric method 68

Discrete analyzers 126
Disodium phenyl phosphate 93
Distilled water 80
Diuretics 116
Dopamine 153
Double beam
  advantages of 50
  spectrophotometer 50
Dry chemistry 52
Dubin Johnson's syndrome 89
Dye excretion test 139
Dyslipidemia 68, 152, 148

## E

Edema 68, 148, 152
Ehrlich's reagent 192
Electrolyte 116, 119
  analysis 113, 114
  estimation of 113
Electrophoresis 108, 111
  apparatus 109f
  principle of 108
  types of 108
Emotional
  disturbances 150
  stress 56
Enzymatic methods 51
Enzyme 121, 173
  ATPase 133
  levels 200
  pancreatic 137
  proteolytic 137
Enzyme-linked immunosorbent
  assay 121, 122f
  indirect 121
  principle 121
  sandwich 122
  types of 121
Epinephrine, degradation of 154
Estrogens 56
Ethereal sulfates 24
  test for 26
Ethylene diamine tetra-acetate 11
Exercise, lack of 81
Extraction, steps of 128
Extrahepatic obstruction 93
Eyes, chemical injury to 9
Fanconi syndrome 85, 97

## F

Fatty acid 160
  essential 161
  monounsaturated 160
  polyunsaturated 160
  saturated 160
  unsaturated 160
Fecal urobilinogen 139
Ferric chloride 69
Filter 114

# Index

First aid
  box 9
  measures 9
Fiske and Subbarow method 84
Flame photometer 113, 114
  components of 114$f$
Fluid deprivation test 146
Folin-Wu method 51, 54, 193
  modified 51, 52
Folin-Wu tube 52, 52$f$
  advantages 52
  reagents required 53
Food
  and glycemic index 157
  energy content of 158
  fats in 160
  glycemic index of 159
Formalin 12
  solution 192
Fouchet's reagent 192
Fouchet's test 31, 32, 135, 144
Fully automated analyzers 126
Functional test meal 134

## G

Galactose metabolism 35, 35$f$
Galactosemia 35, 180
Gallstones 89
Galvanometer 49
Gastric aspiration 120
Gastric function
  assessment of 134
  tests 133
Gastric juice 133, 134, 192
  analysis of 133, 192
    qualitative 134
Gastric mucosa 133
Gastric secretion 134
Gel, preparation of 111
General wastes 10
Gerhardt's test 30
Gilbert's disease 89
Glass electrode 15
Glassware items 6
Globulin 110
  test for 42
Glomerular filtration rate 146, 175
Glomerular function tests 145
Glomerulonephritis, acute 71
Glomerulus acts 145
Glucocorticoids
  excess 153
  functions of 153
  insufficiency of 153
Glucometer 52, 102, 102$f$
Glucose 52
  6 phosphate dehydrogenase
    deficiency 35
  estimation of 42, 51

normal level of 56
oxidase peroxidase 51, 55
standard 193
tolerance, impaired 59, 61$f$
value of 51
Glucose tolerance test 58
  curves 60
  indications 58
  normal 59
  procedure 58
  types of 60
Glycemic index 159
Glycosuria 28
Gmelin's test 31, 144
Goiter 151
Good housekeeping 9
Gout 68, 97, 148, 152, 175
  primary 176
  secondary 176
  types of 176
Gouty arthritis 97
Graves disease 150
Guanine 94

## H

Hay's test 30, 32, 135, 143
Heat coagulation test 29, 32
Heller's test 29, 32
Hematocrits 12
Hematuria 30
Hemoglobin, abnormal 109
Hemoglobinuria 30
Heparin-mucopolysaccharide 11
Hepatic excretory function
  139, 140
Hepatitis
  chronic 91
  viral 89, 91
Hereditary fructose intolerance 36,
  36$f$, 180
Homocystinuria 38, 181
Hormonal disorders 166, 183
Hormones 143, 200
  antidiuretic 146
  thyroid-stimulating 149
Horseradish peroxidase 121
Hot air oven 5
Hyperbilirubinemia
  congenital 89
  conjugated 89
  mixed 89
  unconjugated 89
Hypercalcemia 83
  causes of 83
  symptoms of 84
Hyperchloremia 117
  causes 117
Hypercholesterolemia, familial 181
Hyperglycemia 56

Hyperkalemia 117
  causes 117
Hypernatremia 116
  causes 116
  signs 116
  symptoms 116
Hyperparathyroidism 184
Hyperphosphatemia 85
Hypertension, malignant 71
Hypertensive nephropathy 147
Hyperthyroidism 150
  primary 151
  secondary 151
Hyperuricemia 97
Hypervitaminosis D 85
Hypocalcemia 83
  causes of 83
  symptoms of 83
Hypochloremia 117
  causes 117
Hypocholesterolemia 78
Hypoglycemia 57
Hypokalemia 116
  causes 116
  signs 116
  symptoms 116
  treatment 117
Hyponatremia 116
  causes 116
  signs 116
  symptoms 116
Hypophosphatemia 85
Hypothyroidism 81, 151, 183
  types of 151
Hypouricemia 97
Hypoxanthine 94
Hysterical causes 120
Immunodiffusion 123
  double 124, 124$f$
  principle of 123
  single 124, 124$f$
  technique 124

## I

Immunoelectrophoresis 108
Immunoglobulins 109
Immuodiffusion 123
In vitro tests 149
In vivo tests 149, 150
Infections 56
Inhalation injury 9
Inherited diseases, congenital 57
Inherited disorders 166, 179
Inner reticularis 152
Inorganic sulfates, test for 26
Intracranial diseases 56
Iodoacetate 12
Ion-selective electrode 114, 115, 115$f$
Isoelectric focussing 108

Isoenzyme 92, 109, 173
  carcino-placental 92
Isopropanol 80

## J
Jaffe's method 64
Jaffe's reaction 62, 66, 194
  based on 62
Jaffe's test 27
Jaundice 68, 148, 152, 168
  classification of 88
  hemolytic 169
  hepatic 89, 170
  neonatal 169
  obstructive 170
  physiological 169
  posthepatic 89

## K
Ketone bodies 29
  test for 30, 31
Kidney
  failure 120
  function tests 145
Kidney disease
  chronic 174
  types of 71
Kinetic analysis 48
Kjeldahl-Nesslerization method 73
Kwashiorkor 178

## L
Laboratory equipments 4
Laboratory waste disposal 9
Lactic acid, test for 135
Lactose intolerance 179
Lambert's law 45
Lesch-Nyhan syndrome 97
Leukemia 97
Leukocyte 92
  alkaline phosphatase 92
Levy Jenning's chart 17
Light, source of 49
Lipid 105
  derived 160
  estimation of 140
  metabolism 181
  profile 79
  simple 160
Litmus paper 14
Liver 139
  cancer of 91
  cirrhosis 110
  disease 68, 137, 139, 142, 148, 152, 168
    chronic 110
    metabolic 140
  enzymes, estimation of 141

failure 120
function tests 139, 140
injury 91
  markers of 139, 141
Lloyd's reagent 65
Locate radial artery 119f
Lowery's method 73
Lundh test 138
Lung diseases 120

## M
Maclean's test 135
Macrocytic anemia 178
Malloy and Evelyn method 87
Mancini
  procedure 123
  technique 124
Maple syrup urinary disease 38, 38f
Measuring cylinders 7
Mercuric sulfate 192
Metabolic acidosis 120, 167, 171
Metabolic alkalosis 120, 171
Metabolic disorders 166
Metabolism, inborn errors of 34, 179
Metallic electrode 104
Methionine metabolism 39f
Methylene-bis-acrylamide 111
Microalbuminuria 147
Middle fasciculata 152
Millon's reagent 191
Mixing chamber 126
Molisch's reagent 191
Monochromatic light 47
Monochromators 49
Multiple myeloma 83, 124
Myeloid leukemia, chronic 92
Myocardial infarction 68, 91, 148, 152, 173
Myxedema 151

## N
Nebulizer 113
Nephrotic syndrome 68, 110, 148, 152, 174
Neurosyphilis 42
Night blindness 176
Ninhydrin reagent 191
Non-protein nitrogenous
  substances, test for 192
Noradrenaline 153
Norepinephrine 153
Normal urine 21, 22, 32, 192
  appearance 21
  chemical characteristics 23
  color 21
  odor 22
  physical characteristics 21
  specific gravity 22

specimen collection 21
test for 192
volume 22
Nyctalopia 176

## O
Oakley Fulthorpe
  procedure 123
  technique 124
Oliguria 22, 174
Optical density 46
Optoelectronic instruments 126
Oral contraceptives 116
Organic constituents 24
Osmolality, measurement of 146
Osteomalacia 93
O-toluidine
  method 193
  reagent 193
Ouchterlony double diffusion 123
Oudin
  procedure 123
  technique 124
Output tube 114
Over skin 9
Oxalates 12
Oxygen, reduction of 119

## P
Paget's disease 83, 93
Pancreas, indirect stimulation of 138
Pancreatic amylase 137
Pancreatic exocrine function tests 137
Pancreatic function
  assessment of 137
  tests 137
Pancreatitis 68, 137, 139, 142, 148, 152
  chronic 81
Pandy's test 42
Paper chromatography 105, 106f
  principle 105
  technique 106
Paper electrophoresis 109
  clinical significance 110
  technique 109
Parathyroid disorder 184
Paucialbuminuria 147
Pentagastrin stimulation test 134
Peptic cells 133
Pettenkofer's test 30, 143
pH 13, 23, 143
  determination of 14
  electrometric of 15, 103
  estimation of 13, 14
pH meter 14f, 103, 103f
  operation of 15, 104
  parts of 15, 103
  using 14

# Index

Phenol solution 55
Phenolphthalein indicator 192
Phenylketonuria 36, 36f, 182
Phosphate 24
  buffer 13
Phospholipids 84
Phosphomolybdic acid 53
  reagent 193
Phosphorus, estimation of 84
Phosphotungstic acid reagent 194
Photoelectric colorimeter 46, 46f
Pipettes 7
Placental isoenzyme 93
Plasma
  lipid profile 79
  proteins
    methods of estimation of 73
    methods of fractionation of 73
    synthesis of 139
Point of care testing 101
  advantages 101
  tests 102
Polyacrylamide gel electrophoresis 108, 109, 111
  advantages 112
  applications 112
  procedure 111
Polyenoic acid 160
Polyuria 22
Postrenal causes 71
Potassium 116, 119
  analysis of 114
  iodide 74
Pregnancy, toxemia of 97
Prerenal causes 71
Protein 28
  analysis of 42
  electrophoresis 108
  estimation of 139
  metabolism, congenital disorders of 36
  standard 194
  test for 29, 32, 191
Protein-energy malnutrition 178
Protein-free filtrate 64, 70, 96
  preparation of 53, 62, 69
  readymade 54
Proteinuria 68, 147, 148, 152
  false 29
  functional 29
  glomerular 147
  organic 29
  types of 29
Pseudohyperkalemia 117
  treatment 117
Psoriasis 97
Pump, proportioning 126
Purine metabolism 175

## Q
Quality control 16
  charts 17
  external 16
  internal 16
Quantitative experiments 43

## R
Radioimmunoassays 122
Random access analyzer 126
Reagent 189
  preparation 191
  required 54
Reducing sugar, test for 28
Reference calomel electrode 15
Reinhold's biuret method 75
Reitman and Frankel method 90
Renal causes 71
Renal diseases 97, 174
Renal failure 68, 71, 148, 152
  chronic 116
Renal function tests 145
Renal glycosuria 59, 60f
Renal threshold 147
Renal tubular acidosis 116
Renal tubules 146
Residual phosphorus 84
Resin uptake test 150
Respiratory acidosis 120, 172
Respiratory alkalosis 120, 172
Respiratory quotient 157
Rickets 93, 177
Rothera's mixture 192
Rothera's test 30, 31
Ryle's tube 133

## S
Saturated fats 160
Schiff's test 27
Scurvy 177
Seliwanoff's reagent 191
Serum 80, 91, 94, 116, 121, 200
  alanine aminotransferase 139
  albumin, estimation of 74
  alkaline phosphatase 92, 139, 141
    estimation of 92
  aspartate aminotransferase 139, 141
  bilirubin 87, 139
  calcium
    and phosphorus 82
    estimation of 82
  electrophoretogram, normal 110f
  estimation of 62
  gamma glutamyl transferase 141
  gastrin level 134
  glutamate
    oxaloacetate transaminase 90
    pyruvate transaminase 90
  lipoproteins 109
  phosphorus, estimation of 84
  plasma proteins, estimation of 74
  potassium in 114
  proteins 73
    electrophoretogram of 110
    separation of 109
  total cholesterol in 77
  total proteins, estimation of 73
  transaminases 90
    estimation of 90
  uric acid 94
    estimation of 94
Simmond's disease 57
Single beam 50
  spectrophotometer 49
Smokers, chronic 92
Sodium 119
  analysis of 114
  estimation of 114
  fluoride 12
  hydroxide 74
  hypobromite reagent 192
  nitrite 191
  potassium tartrate 74
  tungstate 193, 194
Solid phase tests 52
Specific dynamic action 158
Spectrophotometer 49f
  applications of 50
  parts 49
  principles of 49
  types 49
Standard solution, preparation of 114
Starch, iodine test for 134
Stick tests 68
Stock ferric chloride reagent 77
Stock solution 194
Stomach, functions of 133
Stroke 120
Sulfates 24
Sulfosalicylic acid 32, 192
  test 29
Sulphanilic acid 192
Sweat electrolytes, estimation of 138
Synthetic function 139, 140

## T
Tandem mass spectrometry 34
Tartaric acid 53
Test tubes 6
Tetraenoic acid 160
Tetraiodothyronine 148
Tetramethylbenzidine 121
Thermogenesis, diet induced 158

Thin layer chromatography 107
Thiosemicarbazide 69, 193
Thymol 12
Thyroid
  antibodies 149, 150
  binding proteins 150
  disorder 148, 152, 183
  function tests 148, 149
  gland 148
  hormones 148
    metabolic effects of 149
    normal values of 148
    unbound 150
  iodine uptake test 150
  scanning 150
  secretion, stimulation of 149
Thyroid-binding globulin 150
Thyrotoxicosis 83
Thyroxine 148
Toluene 12
Topfer's indicator 192
Total bilirubin 87, 88
Total calcium in serum, methods of estimation of 82
Total cholesterol, estimation of 77
Total plasma proteins 140
Total protein, estimation of 194
Total quality management 17
Trans-fatty acids 161
Triacylglycerol 80, 160
Trienoic acid 160
Triglyceride 79, 80, 160
Triiodothyronine 148
Trypsin 137
Tubular functions tests 146
Tumors, treatment of malignant 97
Tungstic acid reagent 195

## U

Uffleman's reagent 192
Uffleman's test 135
Ulcerative colitis 92
Unsaturated fats 160
Urea 24
  clearance 72
  estimation of 68, 70, 193
  standard 194
  structure of 68
  test for 26
Urease
  suspension 192
  test, specific 26
Uremia 71
Uric acid 24, 94-96
  decreased level of 97
  estimation of 94, 96, 194
  increased 97
  methods of estimation of 94
  normal 176
  standard 195
  test for 26
Urinary acidification test 147
Urinary chloride
  decreased 23
  increased 23
Urine 34, 37, 39, 116, 179, 180
  abnormal 22, 32
    chemical constituents of 28
  analysis of 19, 145
    abnormal 31
    normal 25
  bile pigments 139
  centrifuged sediment of 145
  collection of 12
  composition of normal 25
  concentration test 146
  constituents of normal 23
  creatinine in 62, 66, 146
  dipstick test 102
  normal 21, 22, 32, 192
  phosphate in 147
  screening of 34
  sodium in 147
  specific gravity of 146
  sugar in 40
  test for abnormal 192
  urea excretion in 71
Urobilinogen 25, 31
  test for 27, 31

## V

Vacutainer 8
Van den Bergh test 140
Vanillyl mandelic acid 154
Vitamin
  A deficiency 176
  $B_{12}$ deficiency 178
  C deficiency 177
  D deficiency 85
  K deficiency 140
Volumetric flasks 7
Vomiting 116
  prolonged 120
von Gierke's disease 57

## W

Waste, type of 10
Water bath 5
Weighing balances 4
Westgard's multirule chart 17
White blood cells
  lysis of 129
  separation of 129
Wilson's disease 97
Working ferric chloride reagent 77

## X

Xanthine 94

## Z

Zak's method 77
Zero optic density 47
Zone electrophoresis 108